SCREENING FOR COLORECTAL CANCER WITH COLONOSCOPY

Edited by **Rajunor Ettarh**

Screening for Colorectal Cancer with Colonoscopy
http://dx.doi.org/10.5772/59736
Edited by Rajunor Ettarh

Contributors

Carlos Eduardo Pinzón-Florez, Diana Marcela Diaz Quijano, Oscar Andres Gamboa-Garay, Humberto Sifuentes, Rotimi Ayoola, Hamza Abdulla, Evan Brady, Muhammed Sherid, Jorge Bernal, Francisco Javier Sánchez Pujadas, Gloria Fernández-Espárrach, Cristina Rodríguez De Miguel, Jigar Bhagatwala, Arpit Singhal, Subbaramiah Sridhar, Summer Aldrugh, Camille Thelin, Parth Parekh, Sanjay Sikka

Published by InTech

Janeza Trdine 9, 51000 Rijeka, Croatia

Publishing Process Manager Iva Lipovic

Technical Editor InTech DTP team

Cover InTech Design team

First published December, 2015

Printed in Croatia

Additional hard copies can be obtained from orders@intechopen.com

Screening for Colorectal Cancer with Colonoscopy, Edited by Rajunor Ettarh

p. cm.

ISBN 978-953-51-2225-8

For EU product safety concerns:
IN TECH d.o.o., Prolaz Marije Krucifikse Kozulić 3, 51000 Rijeka, Croatia,
info@intechopen.com or visit our website at intechopen.com.

Meet the editor

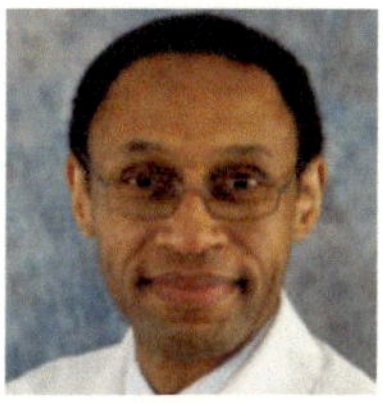

Dr. Rajunor Ettarh is Professor and Vice-Chair for Education in the Department of Structural and Cellular Biology at Tulane University School of Medicine, where he also serves as Director of the Graduate Program in Anatomy. A Fellow of the Royal Society of Medicine in London, he spent much of his research career in Ireland, where his main interests centered on radiobiology and epithelial cell biology of the digestive tract, the regulatory mechanisms that mediate uninhibited proliferation in gastrointestinal cancers, and potential therapeutic targets. He has published extensively, has previously edited two books on colorectal cancer, and reviews for a number of cancer journals.

Contents

Preface

Colorectal cancer remains a major health issue for many developed regions around the world. The good news is that early detection has significantly improved overall survival rates and continues to do so. A number of prevention strategies contribute to this positive trend – all of which are presented and discussed in this series of chapters. What are the risks? The risks are not good: a 5% risk of being diagnosed with colorectal cancer in one's lifetime. The odds are however getting better: 5-year survival rates of up to 90% if the disease is discovered early. For those with predisposing risk factors such as family history, inflammatory bowel disease or adenomatous polyposis, surveillance is recommended.

Surveillance guidelines outlined by several organizations are presented in detail in this book. Whether the aim is to prevent colorectal cancer or to detect the disease early, the role of fecal occult blood tests as well as inspections of the colon by flexible sigmoidoscopy and colonoscopy have been extensively studied and reported. Modalities include programmatic screening of target populations as well as opportunistic tests of patients. What about outcomes? Measured around incidence and mortality, screening remains cost effective, although its value continues to be debated. The issue of interval colorectal cancer remains a challenge. The role that modalities such as computed tomographic colonoscopy and genetic stool testing play in prevention and detection will only become clearer with more data and evidence. Today, a patient who undergoes a colonoscopy for screening purposes stands a much better chance of being effectively surveyed for prevention of colorectal cancer. Patients can rely increasingly on the improved datasets and technical advances that are being made in colonoscopic equipment and skills. The future of surveillance looks increasingly positive as long as progress continues, particularly in the partnership between clinicians and computer scientists, for the development of better tools and methods.

ACKNOWLEDGMENTS

This book would not have been possible without the support of my family. I am also especially indebted to process managers Ivona Lovrić and Iva Lipović whose immense patience, timely reminders, and constant assistance and support made the task of editing this book easier.

Dr. Rajunor Ettarh
Tulane University, School of Medicine,
New Orleans, LA, USA

Section 1

Screening with Colonoscopy

Chapter 1

Colonoscopy Screening for Colorectal Cancer — Overview of the Literature

Carlos Eduardo Pinzon-Florez, Oscar Andres Gamboa-Garay and Diana Marcela Diaz-Quijano

Additional information is available at the end of the chapter

http://dx.doi.org/10.5772/61851

Abstract

Objective: The aim of our chapter was to perform a systematic review of the clinical practice guidelines, randomized clinical trials, and prospective studies, using total colonoscopy for screening this population for colorectal cancer (CRC) and to evaluate the effectiveness of diagnosis and safety.

Methods: We included clinical practice guidelines, systematic reviews, and primary studies with more than 25 participants, and only those reporting the evaluation of colonoscopy as screening test for colorectal cancer and adenoma were included in this chapter. Analysis was performed for three outcomes: accuracy of colonoscopy as a screening test, reduction of colorectal cancer incidence and prevalence, and identification of adverse events of the procedure.

Results: For screening colonoscopy, evidence was of moderate quality. The evidence results suggest tentatively an even stronger reduction in distal colorectal cancer incidence and mortality. The colonoscopy significantly reduces the mortality for CRC. These studies suggest a 17% to 30% lower risk of incident colorectal cancer and 64% death from colorectal cancer after screening colonoscopy vs other screening diagnosis tests.

Conclusions: Colonoscopy is a feasible and safe method for screening CRC for proximal locations in asymptomatic people; however, these findings must be in contrast with the cost of the procedure, accessibility opportunities, and complications.

Keywords: Colonoscopy, Screening, Colorectal cancer, Adenoma, Fecal occult blood test (MeSH terms)

1. Introduction

1.1. Epidemiology of colorectal cancer

1.1.1. The colorectal cancer worldwide

Colorectal cancer is a disease typical of the regions with the largest urban and industrial development, which has changed consumption patterns and life. Worldwide, the rate of age-adjusted incidence (APR) of 17.2 cases per 100,000, ranking fourth in incidence among all types of cancer in both sexes, is presented, with a higher incidence rate in men than in women, APR of 20.3 and 14.6 cases per 100,000, respectively, for a total of 663,000 cases in men and 571,000 cases in women (1). About 60% of these cases occur in developed regions; the highest incidence rates are found in Australia, New Zealand, and Western Europe and the lowest in Africa (excluding South Africa) and South-Central Asia, with intermediate rates in Latin America (1).

Worldwide, the mortality rate adjusted for age (TAE) of colorectal cancer is 8.2 cases per 100,000, being the fifth leading cause of cancer death in both sexes, following lung, breast, stomach, and liver cancer. In men, it is 9.6 cases per 100,000 and for women, it is 7.0 cases per 100,000 (being the fourth most common type in both men and women). Nearly 608,000 deaths per year from colorectal cancer are presented, accounting for 8% of all cancer deaths. Unlike the cases of incidence, the highest mortality rates in both sexes are presented in Central and Eastern Europe (20.1 per 100,000 for men, 12.2 per 100,000 for women) and lower mortality rates are presented in Central Africa (3.5 per 100,000 for men and 2.7 per 100, 000 for women) (1).

The diagnosis is made predominantly with the location of polyps, 92% of them in situ and 40 % of cases are diagnosed at 60 years of age, 30 % at 50, and 30 % at 70. The rest 95 % of diagnoses shows adenocarcinoma type as the predominant pathology, being 80 % of sporadic nature, over the diagnosis of hereditary familial problem like. Less than 3% of patients are under 40 years (2).

Colon and rectal cancer have been associated with various risks, such as chronic ulcerative colitis; sclerosing cholangitis; certain inherited problems; a number of aspects related to eating habits, such as low-residue diet rich in saturated fats, diabetes, obesity, lack of physical activity, low intake of fruits and vegetables, smoking, and alcohol intake; ethnicity; and other genetic factors. However, only age has been measured in quantitative terms to establish the burden attributable to mortality. It is also necessary to specify, through additional studies, the burden of risk factors such as familial adenomatous polyposis, hereditary polypoid colorectal cancer, inflammatory bowel disease, sclerosing cholangitis, and others (2, 3).

Due to many factors, probably related to health technologies and early detection of the problem, among others, in the last 20 years, overall survival increased from 42 to 62 %. According to data in Globocan 2008, the five-year survival can be 72 % in men and 61 % in women (1, 2).

1.2. Colonoscopy and screening

For about two decades, multiple reports of epidemiological studies have concluded that the introduction of endoscopic procedures is effective for strippage of premalignant lesions. The number of countries that have included colonoscopy and sigmoidoscopy as screening strategies for CRC has increased; however, the cost of implementation and potential adverse events limited its use for those in the middle- and low-income population (1-3).

It is clear that in populations at high risk of colorectal cancer (hereditary familial polyposis, ulcerative colitis or Crohn's disease), the screening test of choice is colonoscopy (4-5). Likewise in early detection in the general population, testing fecal occult blood is implemented and after a positive result, confirmatory colonoscopy and treatment is performed, which seeks to remove the precancerous lesion or cancer in situ. Colonoscopy does not fully meet the criteria on being a screening test for CRC because it is expensive; however it has some advantages because it can include treatment of polyp lesions and early cancer; unfortunately, only few studies of controlled trials have been conducted to analyze the performance of colonoscopy as a screening test for CRC. With regard to sigmoidoscopy, the advantages presented are the evaluation of the proximal colon, and only sigmoidoscopy can assess the distal colon, where most cancers occur [6]. Compared to testing fecal occult blood, colonoscopy has a major role in terms of reducing the incidence and mortality of CRC (7); Winawer and colleagues demonstrated a decrease in CRC incidence – 70 to 90 % – in a cohort of 1400 patients after polypectomy compared with controls based on symptoms and physical examination (8,9). In a study in Olmsted County, a decline in annual mortality of 25.2/100,000 to 21.4/100,000 followed the increase at subsequent rate of polypectomies (10).

The objective of this chapter is to review the literature and make some conclusion about total colonoscopy for screening CRC and the complication rate of screening colonoscopy in this setting, particularly bleeding, perforation, and death.

2. Methods

The purpose of this review is to evaluate the effectiveness and safety of colonoscopy as a screening test for adenoma, advanced adenoma, and colorectal cancer. For safety outcome, we evaluated bleeding, perforation, and death.

An asymptomatic person is defined as a person over 40 years and less than 75 years old without abdominal pain, rectal bleeding, weight loss, or changes in bowel habits.

Early and late adenomas were defined as adenomas smaller than 10 mm and greater than 10 mm, respectively, both of villous adenoma histology or high-grade dysplasia.

2.1. Data source and search strategy

We made a literature search in MEDLINE, EMBASE, the Cochrane Library, CINAHL, and LILACS from 1966 to February 2015. On the other hand, we made a search of guidelines in the websites of the developer groups NICE, New Zealand Group, SIGN, North America Centers, IETS in Colombia, and CENETEC in Mexico, using the following keywords: ''screening colonoscopy,'' "colonoscopy," "colorectal cancer," "polyps," and ''screening colorectal cancer.'' The types of secondary studies were systematic reviews of the literature and clinical practice guidelines. The primary study types were controlled clinical trial, observational cohort, and case-control studies. Studies published in Spanish and English were the only ones selected. Likewise, additional searches were made from bibliographies of studies identified in the initial search.

2.2. Study selection

The clinical practice guidelines that were rated with 2 older AGREE (11) 60% quality in the domain of methodology were included. Systematic reviews of the literature described colonoscopy as a screening strategy. For primary studies such as controlled trials and observational analytical studies of moderate to high quality, we included the checklists of SIGN (12).

Exclusion criteria was studies evaluating colonoscopy in high-risk population of CRC, other studies evaluating screening tests without comparison with colonoscopy, likewise studies that do not contemplate the outcomes of interest for this chapter and not to report measures were considered effect with confidence intervals

3. Results

3.1. Evidence that exists for screening colorectal cancer

Screening is the examination of asymptomatic individuals or healthy individuals in order to classify them as likely or unlikely to have a disease (6).

The standard screening test is colonoscopy, but there are alternatives such as flexible sigmoidoscopy, computed tomography colonography (CTC or virtual colonoscopy) (7), fecal occult blood test (FOBT) or stool analysis, and also, evidenced by the literature, combined sigmoidoscopy and FOBT; the alternatives also include barium enema and endoscopy capsule; however, there are insufficient epidemiological studies that support these types of screening (8-15).

The optimal strategy of screening for colorectal cancer is selected considering the following criteria: age of onset and age range in individuals at average risk for this condition.

3.2. Volume of evidence

For this issue, three clinical practice guidelines were included that scored highly in methodology dimension with the AGREE2 checklist: quality assurance in colorectal cancer screening and diagnosis of the IARC (5) Screening for Colorectal Cancer, US Preventive Services Task Force (USPSTF) recommendation statement (17), and a clinical practice guideline for the early detection, diagnosis, treatment, following, and rehabilitation of patients with colorectal cancer of the Colombian Ministry of Health (18).

The review process identified 22 systematic reviews of which six were contained in guidelines previously described (19-24). Of the 16 remaining systematic reviews, two publications were discarded because they did not have clarity in the average-risk population (25; 26) and five for lack of data for the average-risk population (27-31).

The remaining nine studies were scored with the GRADE system. According to screening strategies, four publications analyzed fecal occult blood test (32-35) and two conducted a systematic review of colonoscopy (36), two studies evaluated colonoscopy and compared it with CTC (virtual colonoscopy) (37; 38) and another study evaluated only the CTC (39), and the last review examined capsule endoscopy (40). The American GPC (17) includes a strategy of screening using FOBT, sigmoidoscopy, or colonoscopy beginning at age 50 and ending at age 75.

3.3. Colonoscopy

Colonoscopy is undoubtedly useful in the case of positive fecal occult blood test. The European guide (16) describes that there is limited evidence on the effectiveness of colonoscopy screening to reduce colorectal cancer incidence and mortality. Recent studies suggest that colonoscopy may not be as effective in the right colon and in other segments of the colon and rectum. It also indicates that there is limited evidence suggesting that the interval for colonoscopy should be less than 10 years and may even extend to 20 years. The American guide includes colonoscopy as one method of screening for patients with a 10-year interval (17).

Three of the nine appointed guides as a strategy to colonoscopy screening at intervals of 10 years (18, 22, 24). These recommendations on the ability of colonoscopy as a screening strategy in asymptomatic individuals are not supported by controlled clinical trials; only case-control studies suggest that colonoscopy screening is associated with a low incidence of colorectal cancer (OR 0.46 95 % CI: 0.36.9 to 0.57) and that it decreases colorectal cancer mortality (OR 0.44: 95 % CI: 0.31 to 0.62) (13). The Australian guide suggests that for diagnostic confirmation, in the presence of a positive fecal occult blood test, colonoscopy is indicated, in order to perform biopsies of lesions and therapeutic removal of adenomas (20). The meta-analysis of Niv et al. (38) included ten prospective cohort studies with a total of 68,324 participants in which the procedure was completed by 97%. Colorectal cancer was found in 0.78 % of cases (95 % CI: 0.13 to 2.97): 77 % of CRC patients were in stages I and II. Advanced adenomas occurred in 5 % of cases (95 % CI 4–6 %).

The study of Niv et al. (38), found during the update, concludes that colonoscopy is a feasible method of screening for average-risk individuals; however, the GRADE rating was low for all three outcomes reported: colorectal cancer screening, drilling complications, and bleeding complications because the authors did not present the search strategy. The primary results are contradictory, and no evidence of homogeneity is presented. The study of Brenner Hermann et al. (6) includes four randomized clinical trials, eight case-control studies, and four cohort studies; the result for randomized clinical trial studies reports reduction in overall colorectal cancer mortality in 22–31 %; in meta-analysis, the pooled risk reduction for incidence was estimated to be 18 % (CI 95 % 11–25%) and for mortality from colorectal cancer 28 % (CI 95 % 20–35 %). The result of observational studies for distal colorectal cancer was strong in reduced incidence and mortality, reduction of 64 % (CI 95 % 50–74 %) in incidence colorectal rates and 66 % (38–81 %) in reduced mortality rates for cancer (6). In this study, it was shown that colonoscopy is much more effective in reducing the incidence and mortality of distal colorectal cancer.

Complications were analyzed in five studies, with the following results: piercing, 0.01 % (95 % CI 0.006 to 0.02) and bleeding, 0.05 % (95 % CI: 0.02 to 0.09). No studies evaluating the effectiveness of virtual colonoscopy in reducing colorectal cancer mortality (13, 24, 40) were found.

3.4. Sigmoidoscopy and colonoscopy

The Colombian guide (18) indicates that screening with flexible sigmoidoscopy and colonoscopy can reduce mortality, and both strategies – sigmoidoscopy and colonoscopy – would fare as diagnostic tools. The European GPC appoints only sigmoidoscopy as the strategy to reduce the incidence and mortality when this strategy is part of an organized screening program.

3.5. Computed tomography colonography (virtual colonoscopy) versus colonoscopy

Pickhardt and colleagues (37) evaluated the sensitivity of CTC and colonoscopy for the detection of colorectal cancer. The research group indicates that although most studies argue that the test performance can be improved in line with the prevalence of the disease, the sensitivity of CTC remained independent of the prevalence. The evaluation of the quality design of this study was low in all outcomes, through the use of a single database and in relation to the population, including only two studies of the average-risk population and age higher than 50 years; in addition, the evidence is indirect. The evidence presented by the Blue Cross and Blue Shield Association (39) was rated low because it only included two studies of individuals at average risk and a description of their results does not show confidence intervals. The study of El-Maraghi (40) lacks clear criteria for inclusion and description of homogeneity tests, key in systematic reviews.

3.6. Capsule endoscopy versus colonoscopy

The objective of the study from the Medical Advisory Secretariat (41) was to determine the effectiveness and safety of capsule endoscopy in identifying colorectal cancer and adenomatous polyps in the average-risk population greater than 50 years old and as a screening strategy. They conclude that although capsule endoscopy is a noninvasive method and has lower sensitivity and specificity and accuracy than colonoscopy, its ability in detecting colorectal cancer has not been studied. The qualifying result of the outcomes of sensitivity, specificity, detection of polyps greater than or equal to 6 mm, and detection of any polyp independent of size was low due to the lack of reporting of homogeneity tests.

3.7. Screening intervals

The European guide (16) indicates that in the case of choosing colonoscopy because of the prevalence, there is a case for screening individuals under age 50 or adults over 75 years or more, due to comorbidities that may outweigh the benefits of the examination. The American guide (42) supported this age of completion of screening; it believes that screening can be studied in the age range of 76–84 years and recommends its accomplishment in individuals 85 years or older.

4. Discussion

For colonoscopy screening test, the meta-analysis of Niv et al. (38), performed with cohort studies, suggests that colonoscopy is a possible and desirable CRC screening method in asymptomatic individuals; however, it is not clearly described how the critical evaluation of the articles was performed nor how the reference to the possible publication bias is made. Colonoscopy no randomized controlled trials that indicate the incidence and mortality from colorectal cancer. Evidence from observational studies suggests that this test could reduce the incidence and mortality from colorectal cancer, according to the National Polyp Study (43, 44) and the Italian multicenter study (45), and although it is a highly sensitive technique (26), the evidence is insufficient to exclude or include colonoscopy as the first-line screening strategy (17,25,41). As an additional point, colonoscopy requires specific training by the clinician, is more expensive than other screening tests, presents greater risk of complications during the test, and increases the likelihood of injury in cases in which polypectomy is performed.

Virtual colonoscopy is a highly specific test, particularly for polyps <9mm; however, the sensitivity varies widely, even for large polyps. The low efficiency of studies to explain the variability of the sensitivity requires rethinking and further study of this test, before recommending it for everyday use in the assessment of polyps (46).

Sigmoidoscopy, colonoscopy, barium enema, and even virtual colonoscopy are up-to-date diagnostic tools for which a greater number of studies evaluating the effectiveness of these methods as the primary screening tests in asymptomatic persons are required (13, 24, 42).

There is a possible overrepresentation of the state of health of the people attending for colonoscopy in analytical observational studies, which may incur information bias. Furthermore, it is possible confounding by these context variables that influence the development of a colonoscopy as well as the incidence of CRC, such as family history, diet, and physical activity.

5. Conclusion

We conclude that colonoscopy may be offered as a CRC screening tool for the high-risk population as well as the asymptomatic population since the diagnostic yield for polyps and cancer is high. These results have to be evaluated with further research and weighed against the cost, accessibility, quality of life of patients, and possible serious complications.

Author details

Carlos Eduardo Pinzon-Florez[1*], Oscar Andres Gamboa-Garay[1,2] and Diana Marcela Diaz-Quijano[1]

*Address all correspondence to: carlos.pinzon1@unisabana.edu.co

1 Health Research Group. Universidad de La Sabana, Colombia

2 Analyses Research Group. National Cancer Institute. Bogota, Colombia

References

[1] Smith RA, Cokkinides V, Brooks D, Saslow D, Brawley OW. Cancer screening in the United State, 2010: a review of current American Cancer Society guidelines and issues in cancer screening. CA Cancer J Clin. 2010;60(2):90-119. Review.

[2] Brown ML, Riley GF, Schussler N, Etzioni R. Estimating health care costs related to cancer treatment from SEER-Medicare data. Med Care. 2002;40(8 Suppl):IV-104-17.

[3] Parkin DM, Whelan SL, Ferlay J, Teppo L, Thomas DB, editors. Cancer incidence in five continents. Vol. VIII. Lyon: International Agency for Research on Cancer; 2002.

[4] Ries LAG, Melbert D, Krapcho M, Stinchcomb DG, Howlader N, Horner M, et al., editors. SEER Cancer Statistics Review, 1975-2005 [Internet]. Bethesda: National Cancer Institute; 2008 [Citado: 29 diciembre 2009]. Disponible en: http://seercancer gov/ csr/ 1975_2005/ 2008.

[5] Ferlay J, Bray F, Pisani P, Parkin DM. GLOBOCAN 2002: Cancer Incidence, Mortality and Prevalence Worldwide [computer program]. IARC Cancer Base No. 5, version 2,0. Lyon: IARC Press; 2004.

[6] Brenner H, Stock C, Hoffmeister M. Effect of screening sigmoidoscopy and screening colonoscopy on colorectal cáncer incidence and mortality: systematic Review and meta-analysis of randomised controlled trials and observational studies. BMJ. 2014;48:g2467.

[7] Winawer SJ, Fletcher RH, Miller L, Godlee F, Stolar M, Mulrow CD, et al. Colorectal cancer screening: clinical guidelines and rationale. Gastroenterology. 1997;112(2): 594-642.

[8] Tsai CJ, Lu DK. Small colorectal polyps: histopathology and clinical significance. Am J Gastroenterol. 1995;90(6):988-94.

[9] Eide TJ. Natural history of adenomas. World J Surg. 1990;15(1):3-6.

[10] Stryker SJ, Wolff BG, Culp CE, Libbe SD, Ilstrup DM, MacCarty RL. Natural history of untreated colonic polyps. Gastroenterology. 1987;93(5):1009-13.

[11] AGREE Collaboration. Appraisal of guidelines for research & evaluation (AGREE) instrument [Internet]. London: The AGREE Collaboration; 2001 [Citado: 24 noviembre 2008]. 22 p. Disponible en: http://www.agreecollaboration.org/ instrument/.

[12] Scottish Intercollegiate Guidelines Network. SIGN 50: A guideline developer's handbook [Internet]. Edinburgh: SIGN; 2008 [Citado: 24 noviembre 2008]. 112 p. Disponible en: http://www.sign.ac.uk/guidelines/fulltext/50/ index.html.

[13] Pignone M, Rich M, Teutsch SM, Berg AO, Lohr KN. Screening for colorectal cancer in adults at average risk: a summary of the evidence for the U.S. Preventive Services Task Force. Ann Intern Med. 2002;137(2):132-41. Review.

[14] Imperiale TF, Wagner DR, Lin CY, Larkin GN, Rogge JD, Ransohoff DF. Risk of advanced proximal neoplasms in asymptomatic adults according to the distal colorectal findings. N Engl J Med. 2000;343(3):169-74.

[15] Anderson BO, Braun S, Lim S, Smith RA, Taplin S, Thomas DB, et al. Early detection of breast cancer in countries with limited resources. Breast J. 2003;9 (Suppl 2):S51-9.

[16] Smith RA, Cokkinides V, Eyre HJ; American Cancer Society. American Cancer Society guidelines for the early detection of cancer, 2003. CA Cancer J Clin. 2003;53(1): 27-43.

[17] McLeod RS; Canadian Task Force on Preventive Health Care. Screening strategies for colorectal cancer: a systematic review of the evidence. Can J Gastroenterol. 2001;15(10):647-60.

[18] Minister of Health Colombia. Guidelines for the prevention, early detection and management of Colorectal Cancer (CRC). Colombia, 2012.

[19] National Medical Research Council. Clinical Practice Guideline. Singapore: Singapore Ministry of Health; 2004.

[20] Winawer S, Fletcher R, Rex D, Bond J, Burt R, Ferrucci J, et al. Colorectal cancer screening and surveillance: clinical guidelines and rationale – update based on new evidence. Gastroenterology. 2003;124(2):544-60.

[21] Institute for Clinical Systems Improvement. Health Care Guidelines: Colorectal cancer screening. 11th ed. Bloomington: Institute for Clinical Systems Improvement; 2006.

[22] Whitlock EP, Lin JS, Liles E, Beil TL, Fu R. Screening for colorectal cancer: a targeted, updated systematic review for the U.S. Preventive Services Task Force. Ann Intern Med. 2008;149(9):638-58.

[23] van Rossum LG, van Rijn AF, Laheij RJ, van Oijen MG, Fockens P, van Krieken HH, et al. Random comparison of guaiac and immunochemical fecal occult blood tests for colorectal cancer in a screening population. Gastroenterology. 2008;135(1):82-90.

[24] Valiñas L, Atienza Merino G. Evaluación de la eficacia y efectividad del cribado poblacional del cáncer colorrectal. Aplicabilidad en el Sistema Nacional de Salud. Santiago de Compostela: Servicio Galego de Saúde, Axencia de Avaliación de Tecnoloxías Sanitarias de Galicia, avalia-t; 2002.

[25] Moayyedi P, Achkar E. Does fecal occult blood testing really reduce mortality? A reanalysis of systematic review data. Am J Gastroenterol. 2006;101(2):380-4.

[26] Hewitson P, Glasziou P, Irwig L, Towler B, Watson E. Screening for colorectal cancer using the faecal occult blood test, Hemoccult. Cochrane Database Syst Rev. 2007;(1):CD001216. Review.

[27] Faivre J, Dancourt V, Lejeune C, Tazi M, Lamour J, Gerard D, et al. Reduction in colorectal cancer mortality by fecal occult blood screening in a French controlled study. Gastroenterology. 2004;126(7):1674-80.

[28] Kronborg O, Jørgensen OD, Fenger C, Rasmussen M. Randomized study of biennial screening with a faecal occult blood test: results after nine screening rounds. Scand J Gastroenterol. 2004;39(9):846-51.

[29] Jørgensen OD, Kronborg O, Fenger C. A randomised study of screening for colorectal cancer using faecal occult blood testing: results after 13 years and seven biennial screening rounds. Gut. 2002;50(1):29-32.

[30] Hardcastle JD, Chamberlain JO, Robinson MH, Moss SM, Amar SS, Balfour TW, et al. Randomised controlled trial of faecal-occult-blood screening for colorectal cancer. Lancet. 1996;348(9040):1472-7.

[31] Towler B, Irwig L, Glasziou P, Kewenter J, Weller D, Silagy C. A systematic review of the effects of screening for colorectal cancer using the faecal occult blood test, Hemoccult. BMJ. 1998;317(7158):559-65.

[32] Mandel JS, Church TR, Bond JH, Ederer F, Geisser MS, Mongin SJ, et al. The effect of fecal occult-blood screening on the incidence of colorectal cancer. N Engl J Med. 2000;343(22):1603-7.

[33] Lindholm E, Brevinge H, Haglind E. Survival benefit in a randomized clinical trial of faecal occult blood screening for colorectal cancer. Br J Surg. 2008;95(8):1029-36.

[34] Hol L, Wilschut JA, van Ballegooijen M, van Vuuren AJ, van der Valk H, Reijerink J, et al. Screening for colorectal cancer: random comparison of guaiac and immuno-

chemical faecal occult blood testing at different cut-off levels. Br J Cancer. 2009;100(7):1103-10.

[35] Medical Services Advisory Committee. Faecal occult blood testing for population health screening. MSAC Reference 18. Assessment Report. Canberra: MSAC; 2004.

[36] De Laet C, Neyt M, Vinck I, Lona M, Cleemput I, Van De Sande S. Health Technology Assessment. Colorectale Kankerscreening: wetenschappelijke stand van zaken en budgetimpact voor België. Brussels: Health Technology Assessment (HTA); 2006.

[37] Hoff G, Grotmol T, Skovlund E, Bretthauer M; Norwegian Colorectal Cancer Prevention Study Group. Risk of colorectal cancer seven years after flexible sigmoidoscopy screening: randomised controlled trial. BMJ. 2009;338:b1846.

[38] Niv Y, Hazazi R, Levi Z, Fraser G. Screening colonoscopy for colorectal cancer in asymptomatic people: a metaanalysis. Dig Dis Sci. 2008;53(12):3049-54.

[39] Smith RA, Cokkinides V, Eyre HJ; American Cancer Society. American Cancer Society guidelines for the early detection of cancer, 2004. CA Cancer J Clin. 2004;54(1): 41-52.

[40] Walsh JM, Terdiman JP. Colorectal cancer screening: scientific review. JAMA. 2003;289(10):1288-96.

[41] Mandel JS, Bond JH, Bradley M, Snover DC, Church TR, Williams S, et al. Sensitivity, specificity and positive predictivity of the Hemoccult test in screening for colorectal cancers. The University of Minnesota's Colon Cancer Control Study. Gastroenterology. 1989;97(3):597-600.

[42] Kerr J, Broadstock M, Day P, Hogan S. Effectiveness and cost-effectiveness of population screening for colorectal cancer. A systematic review of the literature. Christchurch, New Zealand: New Zealand Health Technology Assessment; 2005.

[43] Mulhall BP, Veerappan GR, Jackson JL. Meta-analysis: computed tomographic colonography. Ann Intern Med. 2005;142(8):635-50.

[44] Winawer SJ, Stewart ET, Zauber AG, Bond JH, Ansel H, Waye JD, et al. A comparison of colonoscopy and double-contrast barium enema for surveillance after polypectomy. National Polyp Study Work Group. N Engl J Med. 2000;342(24):1766-72.

[45] Citarda F, Tomaselli G, Capocaccia R, Barcherini S, Crespi M; Italian Multicentre Study Group. Efficacy in standard clinical practice of colonoscopic polypectomy in reducing colorectal cancer incidence. Gut. 2001;48(6):812-5.

[46] Prorok PC, Andriole GL, Bresalier RS, Buys SS, Chia D, Crawford ED, et al. Design of the Prostate, Lung, Colorectal and Ovarian (PLCO) cancer screening trial. Control Clin Trials. 2000;21(6 Suppl):273S-309S.

Chapter 2

Screening and Surveillance Colonoscopy

Rotimi R. Ayoola, Hamza Abdulla, Evan K. Brady, Muhammed Sherid and Humberto Sifuentes

Additional information is available at the end of the chapter

http://dx.doi.org/10.5772/61204

Abstract

Colorectal cancer is a major cause of worldwide morbidity and mortality. As such, there are many guidelines and recommendations set forth by various medical societies regarding colonoscopy for screening and surveillance. The universal goal of these guidelines is to reduce colorectal cancer prevalence and mortality. Recommendations for colorectal cancer screening and surveillance using colonoscopy vary slightly between medical society guidelines and are often dictated by some combination of age, known disease severity, length of time since last study, family history, and comorbid conditions.

Keywords: Screening, surveillance, colonoscopy, recommendations, colorectal cancer

1. Introduction

Colorectal cancer is the second leading cause of death from cancer in the United States, as well as the fourth most common cause of cancer-related death, and the third most diagnosed cancer worldwide.[1, 3] In 2008, there were an estimated 1.2 million newly diagnosed cases of colorectal cancer worldwide and an estimated 609,000 colorectal cancer-related deaths.[3] In 2014, it was estimated that there were 136,830 newly diagnosed cases of colorectal cancer and nearly 50,310 deaths associated with this disease in the Unites States alone.[4] The age-adjusted incidence of colorectal cancer in the United States was 43.7 cases per 100,000 population among men and women based on reported cases from 2007 to 2011.[4] In 2011, there were an estimated 1,162,426 people living with colon and rectum cancer in the United States.[4] Screening of those at average risk may result in lower mortality rates by detecting cancers at earlier and more curable stages. Also, detection of cancer-precursor lesions may reduce the incidence of colorectal cancer if removed on endoscopic screening tests.[5, 6] The incidence and mortality of colorectal cancer have declined from 2002 to 2010 in the United States,[7] possibly due to improvement in the adherence to screening and surveillance guidelines.

2. Colorectal cancer screening

2.1. Prevention strategies

Recommended strategies for colorectal cancer screening can be divided into two categories: stool tests (occult blood and DNA tests) and structural examinations (flexible sigmoidoscopy, colonoscopy, double contrast barium enema, capsule endoscopy, and computed tomographic colonography). Each screening method has its own advantages and disadvantages, which are summarized in Table 1. Screening is currently recommended beginning at 50 years of age in average-risk populations, and varies in populations with increased risks.[6, 8]

Test	Advantages	Disadvantages
Sensitive guaiac fecal occult blood test	Inexpensive, easily done at home	Low sensitivity, annually repeated, lack of compliance
Fecal immunochemical test	Inexpensive, easily done at home	More expensive than guaiac fecal occult, annually repeated, unknown adherence, low sensitivity for advanced adenomas
Stool DNA	More accurate than blood detection; easily done at home	Expensive, sensitivity and specificity unknown, uncertain screening intervals
CT Colonography	High sensitivity of lesions >10 mm in diameter; not invasive	Not been proven to reduce incidence or mortality, bowel prep needed, unknown management of polyps <6 mm in diameter, radiation exposure
Sigmoidoscopy	Can be done in office without sedation, 60% reduction in mortality from cancer of the distal colon	Proximal colon cancer may be missed
Colonoscopy	90% sensitivity for lesions >10 mm in diameter, 53-72% reduction in incidence and 31% reduction in mortality from colorectal cancer, lesions can be detected and removed during one examination	Bowel preparation and expertise needed, expensive, invasive with possible complications

**Data from Lieberman[6], Baxter, et al.[9], Muller, et al.[10], and Singh, et al.[11]

Table 1. Advantages and disadvantages of screening tests

http://dx.doi.org/10.5772/61204

Strategies used to identify patients at an increased risk for developing colorectal cancer should be started early. Before determining the best screening tool, clinicians should determine a patient's level of risk. The most common indicator of increased risk is a first-degree relative with colorectal cancer. Diagnosis of colorectal cancer in a first-degree relative before 50 years of age is concerning for hereditary gastrointestinal cancer syndromes such as Lynch syndrome, familial adenomatous polyposis (FAP), attenuated familial adenomatous polyposis (AFAP), and MUTYH-associated polyposis (MAP). Patients with hereditary gastrointestinal cancer syndromes require a special timing for endoscopic screening and surveillance. Colonoscopy is the preferred screening test in these persons, which should be initiated at 40 years of age or 10 years younger than the age at which the family member was diagnosed with colorectal cancer, whichever comes first.[6, 8] Patients with chronic ulcerative colitis or colitis due to Crohn's disease are at increased risk for colorectal cancer and should undergo a screening colonoscopy after 8-10 years.[6, 8] Prior colorectal cancer or polyps also increases the risk of colorectal cancer, especially if polyps are large, or have villous architecture.[12]

2.2. Identifying high-risk individuals

The risk of developing colorectal cancer is largely multifactorial. The factors associated with an increased risk of colorectal cancer include lack of physical activity, obesity, high-fat and low-fiber diets, tobacco use, gender, ethnicity, and genetics. There is limited evidence to suggest that lifestyle modification alone in adults will reduce the risk of this cancer.[6, 13] Aspirin, nonsteroidal anti-inflammatory drugs, and hormone-replacement therapy can decrease the risk of adenomas or colorectal cancer but are not recommended in prevention of colorectal cancer because the possible adverse effects are higher than the potential benefits.[6, 14, 15]

2.3. Screening modalities

Multiple tests are used as options for colorectal cancer screening. Stool-based tests can improve disease prognosis by detecting early cancers. Endoscopic or radiologic tests can visualize the bowel mucosa and detect polyps that can be removed before malignant transformation. Sensitivities of various screening modalities (Table 2) and screening guidelines (Table 3) can be very useful when choosing the most appropriate screening test.

Test	**Sensitivity**		**References**
	Cancer Detection	**Advanced Adenoma* Detection**	
Standard guaiac fecal occult blood test (three stool samples)	33-50%	11%	Mandel et al.[16], Hardcastle et al.[17], Kronborg et al.[18], Imperiale TF.[19], Ahlquist.[20]

Test		Sensitivity	References
Sensitive guaiac fecal occult blood test (three stool samples)	50-75%	20-25%	Allison et al.[15], Levin et al.[21], Whitlock et al.[22], Ahlquist et al.[20]
Immunochemical fecal occult blood test (one-three stool samples)	60-85%	20-50%	Levin et al.[21], Whitlock et al.[22]
Old stool DNA test (one stool sample)	51%	18%	Imperiale et al.[19]
New stool DNA test (one stool sample)	≥80%	40%	Allison et al.[15], Itzkowitz et al.[23]
CT Colonography	Uncertain; probably >90%	90% (if ≥10 mm diameter)	Johnson et al.[24]
Sigmoidoscopy	>95% (for distal colon)	70%	Lieberman[6], Shelby et al.[25]
Colonoscopy	>95%	88-98%	Lieberman[6], Imperiale et al.[19], Schoenfeld et al.[26], Lieberman et al.[27], Pickhardt et al.[28], Cotton et al.[29], Rockey et al.[30]

*Advanced adenoma is defined as tubular adenoma that is ≥10 mm in diameter or with villous histologic features or high-grade dysplasia.

Table 2. Sensitivity of one-time colorectal cancer screening tests

Screening Test	ACS-MSTF-ACR	USPSTF	Recommended Interval for Rescreening
Sensitive guaiac fecal occult blood test	Recommended if "/>50% sensitivity for colorectal cancer	Recommended	1 yr
Fecal immunochemical test	Recommended if >50% sensitivity for colorectal cancer	Recommended; high-sensitivity test only	1 yr
Stool DNA test	Recommended if >50% sensitivity for colorectal cancer	Not Recommended (insufficient evidence to assess sensitivity and specificity of fecal DNA)	Uncertain

Screening Test	ACS-MSTF-ACR	USPSTF	Recommended Interval for Rescreening
Flexible sigmoidoscopy	Recommended if sigmoidoscope is inserted to 40 cm of the colon or to the splenic flexure	Recommended; with guaiac fecal occult blood test every 3 yr	5 yr
Barium enema Examination	Recommended, but only if other tests not available	Not recommended	5 yr
CT colonography	Recommended, with referral for colonoscopy if polyps ≥6 mm in diameter detected	Not recommended (insufficient evidence to determine risk-benefit ratio)	5 yr
Colonoscopy	Recommended	Recommended	10 yr

* Data from Lieberman[6], Preventive Services Task Force[14], Levin et al.[21], Preventive Services Task Force[14], and Whitlock et al.[22]; ACS-MSTF-ACR denotes American cancer Society, US Multisociety task force on Colorectal Cancer, and American College of Radiology; and USPSTF denotes US Preventive services Task Force.

Table 3. US colorectal cancer screening guidelines, 2008*

2.3.1. Fecal screening tests

Fecal screening tests use small stool samples to help determine the presence of colorectal cancer. Fecal screening tests include Guaiac-based fecal occult blood test, immunochemical-based fecal occult blood test, also known as fecal immunochemical test (FIT), and Cologuard (fecal DNA testing, combined with hemoglobin and DNA methylation assays). These tests are easily performed at home or in a clinical office, are noninvasive, inexpensive, without direct adverse health effects, and require few specialized resources. One disadvantage of fecal testing is that positive results require colonoscopy evaluation to confirm or exclude the diagnosis of colorectal cancer.

Guaiac fecal occult blood tests detect hemoglobin peroxidase activity and turn guaiac-impregnated paper blue, but are not specific for human blood. Three separate stool samples per test are preferred for better sensitivity.[21] The fecal occult blood test is associated with significant false-positive results, which may lead to unnecessary follow-up colonoscopies. In the Minnesota trial, false-positive test results were found in almost 9% of fecal occult blood testing.[3] The cost-effectiveness of colorectal cancer screening with an annual or biennial fecal occult blood test varied from US$ 5,691 to US$ 17,805 per life-year gained.[31] Randomized, controlled trials in which standard guaiac tests were administered annually or biennially have shown that cancers are detected at an earlier and more curable stage when compared with no regular screening. Over a period of 10-13 years, regular guaiac screening tests result in a reduction of colorectal cancer mortality by 15-33%.[6, 8, 32]

FIT uses antibodies specific to hemoglobin to screen for colorectal cancer. It is more accurate than the guaiac test.[33, 37] As a result, FIT is now recommended as the first-choice fecal occult blood test in colorectal cancer screening.[38] FIT has sensitivity for detecting cancer of 60-85%

with the use of one to three stool samples.[4, 6, 22] Cologuard is a screening modality that tests stool DNA for specific mutations that are associated with colorectal cancer. These specific segments of cellular DNA are excreted in stool and can be detected with the use of polymerase chain reaction (PCR) amplification. Newer versions of the test are currently being developed; however, overall performance, utility, and cost-effectiveness has not been well studied.

2.3.2. *Structural examinations of the colon*

Colorectal cancers can be detected through physical exams with a digital rectal examination, but there is little evidence to support the effectiveness of digital rectal exam in the detection of colorectal cancer and, therefore, it is not recommended in the current screening guidelines (Table 3).

Anatomical examination of the colon is effective in detection of early cancer and precancerous lesions. Radiography imaging such as barium enema and computed tomographic (CT) colonography can be used to detect lesions. In clinical studies of CT colonography for polyp detection with expert radiologists, 90% of polyps 10 mm or larger in diameter were identified correctly, with a false-positive rate of 14%.[6] CT colonography is not as sensitive for polyps less than 6 mm. There are currently no conclusive studies supporting appropriate screening intervals for negative results or suitable next steps for polyps less than 6 mm. While radiation exposure during CT colonography is considered minimal, the cumulative radiation exposure puts people at increased risk for developing other types of radiation-related cancers. Additionally, cost-effectiveness of CT colonography has not been thoroughly studied in comparison to other modalities.

Before colonoscopy became available, barium enema was the primary means of detecting polyps, and their removal required surgical colostomy.[39] Barium enema examination is not the best test for identifying precancerous lesions and is rarely used for colorectal-cancer screening in current practice.[6] Double-contrast barium enema is another screening modality that involves the patient drinking contrast, which coats the intestinal mucosa with barium. Then, the colon is insufflated with air and multiple radiographs are taken under fluoroscopy. Double-contrast barium enema detects about half of adenomas larger than 1 cm and 39% of all polyps.[40] Retrospective studies have found that double-contrast barium enema failed to diagnose 15-22% of colorectal cancers.[41] If an abnormality is found, then colonoscopy evaluation should follow. False-positives or inconclusive results can be a result of stool, mucosal irregularities, or air. Barium enemas are safe and typically do not require sedation, but may cause the patient discomfort during the procedure. The usage rates of double contrast barium enema for colorectal cancer screening recently declined with improved screening tools, but may be useful where colonoscopy is not readily available.[42]

Endoscopic screening is more sensitive than fecal testing for the detection of adenomatous polyps.[37, 43, 45] In the United Kingdom, one-time screening with flexible sigmoidoscopy significantly reduced the incidence of colorectal cancer by 23% and cancer-related mortality by 31%.[45, 46] Studies, with the use of screening colonoscopy, have shown that more than 30% of patients with advanced neoplasia have proximal lesions that would not be identified with sigmoidoscopy alone.[47, 48]

The most performed indication for colonoscopy in the United States is for screening and surveillance purposes. Colonoscopy can detect a wide range of colon pathologies including polyps, angiodysplasias, hemorrhoids, and cancer. Colonoscopy also permits therapeutic interventions. The procedure is highly feasible and relatively safe. The quality of the procedure depends on an adequate bowel preparation. The patient is typically sedated throughout the procedure. Colonoscopy can reduce the incidence and the mortality of colorectal cancer.[9, 27, 49] Endoscopic procedures may be uncomfortable for patients and carry the risks of perforation and bleeding, especially when polypectomy is performed. The risk of serious adverse events is 3-5 events per 1000 colonoscopies.[6]

Capsule endoscopy has the potential to become a useful screening tool. A camera, in the size and shape of a pill, is swallowed to help visualize the gastrointestinal tract. Reductions of incidence and mortality have not yet been studied using this modality. Capsule endoscopy does not require sedation or radiation. However, accuracy data show inferior screening performance compared to colonoscopy.[3] Despite all these available methods, colorectal cancer screening rates are still suboptimal. In a National Health Interview Survey in 2010, the rate of screening was only 58.6%.[39]

2.4. Screening guidelines

Two major guidelines, from the US Preventive Services Task Force (USPSTF) and a joint guideline from the American Cancer Society, the US Multi-Society Task Force on Colorectal Cancer, and the American College of Radiology (ACS-MSTF), were released in 2008 regarding colorectal cancer screening in the United States (Table 3). The joint guidelines recommend structural examinations for cancer prevention. The ACS-MSTF recommends offering screening beginning at age 50 years for average-risk patients, and continued surveillance every 10 years, if negative. In average-risk patients, CT colonography should be performed every 5 years, flexible sigmoidoscopy every 5 years, and double-contrast barium enema every 5 years. The joint guidelines recommend fecal occult blood testing with sensitive guaiac method or fecal immunochemical-based test every year for screening. Screening should be terminated if a patient's life expectancy is less than 10 years.[21] Prior to screening, patients should understand that a positive test indicates a need for colonoscopy. There are no specific guidelines regarding colorectal cancer screening for sex or ethnicity but the American College of Gastroenterology supports initiation of screening in African Americans at 45 years of age.[8]

The US Preventive Services Task Force does not recommend CT colonography or stool DNA testing. The USPSTF recommends three screening options for adults 50-75 years old: sensitive fecal occult blood testing annually, flexible sigmoidoscopy every 5 years with sensitive fecal occult blood test every 3 years, and colonoscopy every 10 years. Screening for patients older than 75 is not routinely recommended by the USPSTF, and recommends against screening over the age of 85 years.[14] Colorectal cancer screening in older patients who have never undergone formal screening is controversial and there are currently no guidelines regarding appropriate screening in these scenarios. The risk of colorectal cancer and advanced polyps continues to increase in age even after 75 years. Thus, the decision to screen between the ages of 75 and 85 years should be discussed with and individualized to each patient depending on health status and other comorbidities.

In Europe, fecal occult blood testing is implemented at higher rates than in the United States. The fecal occult blood test for individuals aged 50-74 years at average-risk has been recommended to date by the European Union guidelines for colorectal screening, annually or biennially.[15]

The British Society of Gastroenterology (BSG) and the Association of Coloproctology for Great Britain and Ireland (ACPGBI) aimed to provide guidance on the appropriateness, method, and frequency of screening for people at moderate- and high-risk for colorectal cancer.[50]

3. Colorectal cancer surveillance

Surveillance colonoscopy refers to colonoscopy examination performed in asymptomatic individuals with previously identified cancerous or precancerous lesions. Colonoscopy surveillance is used to identify any recurrent or new neoplasia in these individuals.[51] High adenoma detection rate on follow-up colonoscopy (30-50%) provides the rationale for surveillance colonoscopy.[52, 56] There is strong evidence that surveillance colonoscopy decreases colorectal cancer incidence and colorectal cancer-related mortality.[57]

The timing of subsequent surveillance is crucial. Studies demonstrate both the protective effect and cost-effectiveness of performing surveillance colonoscopy on high-risk populations.[58] The overall impact of surveillance is not well defined and may be decreased by an inappropriate utilization of resources and nonadherence to published guidelines.[59]

3.1. Recommendations for surveillance colonoscopy

Guidelines from Gastrointestinal societies in the United States, the United Kingdom, and the European Union follow a risk stratification policy to time their surveillance intervals.

The US Multisociety Task Force (US MSTF) guidelines were published in 2008 and categorize patients into two major risk groups based on the likelihood of development of advanced neoplasia (Table 4). In 2012, the US MSFT updated their guidelines to address the role of serrated polyps, risk of interval colorectal cancer, and proximal colorectal cancer (Table 5).

The European Society of Gastrointestinal Endoscopy (ESGE) updated their guidelines in 2013 and formulated a risk stratification and surveillance strategy similar to the United States (Table 4 and Table 5). A new recommendation was to increase the interval from 3 years to 5 years after a normal follow-up colonoscopy in the high-risk group (3-4 adenomas, villous features or high-grade dysplasia, or ≥10 mm in size).

The UK guidelines are based on adenoma size and number without incorporating histological findings. It stratifies patients into low-, moderate-, and high-risks groups. It also recommends a "single clearing examination" at 1 year for high-risk patients (≥5 small adenomas or ≥3 adenomas, at least 1 of which is ≥1 cm).

	United States Multisociety Task Force (US MSTF)	European Society of Gastrointestinal Endoscopy (ESGE)	British Society of Gastroenterology (BSG)
Risk			
Low	1-2 tubular adenomas <10 mm	1–2 tubular adenomas <10 mm with low-grade dysplasia; serrated polyps < 10 mm and no dysplasia	1–2 adenomas <10 mm
Moderate	-	-	3–4 adenomas <10 mm or at least one adenoma >1cm
High	Adenoma with villous histology or high-grade dysplasia or ≥10 mm or ≥3 adenomas	Adenoma with villous histology or high-grade dysplasia or ≥ 10 mm in size, or ≥3 adenomas; serrated polyps ≥ 10 mm or with dysplasia	>5 small adenomas or at least 3 adenomas >1cm

Table 4. Risk stratification criteria

	United States Multisociety Task Force (US MSTF)	European Society of Gastrointestinal Endoscopy (ESGE)	British Society of Gastroenterology (BSG)
Risk			
Low	5-10 years	10 years	No surveillance or 5 years
Moderate	-	-	3 years
High	**3 years**	3 years	1 years

Table 5. Surveillance interval recommendation

A recently published study, which analyzed 3226 post-polypectomy patients, compared the US MSTF guidelines with the British Society of Gastroenterology (BSG) guidelines. The study showed that the application of the UK guidelines into the US population reclassified 26.3% of patients from high-risk to a higher-risk category and 7% to a lower-risk category.[60] The study also showed a net 19% of patients benefiting from detection 2 years earlier without substantially increasing rates of colonoscopy.[60]

3.2. Sessile serrated adenomas/polyps and surveillance colonoscopy

Sessile serrated adenoma/polyp (SSA/P) is a term used to describe polyps or adenomas characterized by the presence of a sawtooth appearance to crypt contour with prominent dilatation, serrations, and lateralization at the crypt base.[51] The discovery of the serrated adenoma/polyp pathway and the development of colorectal cancer has led to increased interest and focus on the understanding of the histological and molecular changes that lead to CRC. Hypermethylation of genes in serrated lesions leads to microsatellite instability and rapid development of colorectal cancer.[61]

Endoscopically, serrated lesions have a similar appearance to hyperplastic polyps and are often misdiagnosed as such. A recent study showed that as high as one-third of recently diagnosed hyperplastic polyps ≥5 mm were reclassified into SSA/P after a second pathology review.[62] The CARE study found that serrated lesions were five times more likely to be incompletely resected by polypectomy compared to conventional adenomas.[63] Serrated polyps larger than 1 cm or with a dysplastic component are considered advanced polyps.[63]

Surveillance recommendations for serrated adenomas/polyps are inconsistent among researchers and gastrointestinal societies and long-term studies evaluating SSA/P are limited. US MSTF and ESGE classifies serrated polyps <10 mm with no dysplasia as low-risk and serrated polyps ≥10 mm or those with dysplasia as high-risk. Both societies recommend surveillance colonoscopy in 3 years in high-risk. For low-risk lesions, ESGE recommends 10-year follow-up, whereas US MSTF recommends 5-year follow-up.[14, 50, 64]

3.3. Serrated polyposis syndrome

The World Health Organization defines serrated polyposis syndrome by either the presence of five or more serrated polyps proximal to the sigmoid colon (at least two of which must be ≥10 mm) or 20 or more serrated polyps of any size distributed throughout the colon.[65] US MSFT and ESGE recommend one-year follow-up surveillance in this patient population. [14, 66] ESGE also recommends referral for genetic counseling.[14, 66]

3.4. Effect of positive family history on surveillance intervals

Patients with a family history of colorectal carcinoma are at higher risk of developing high-risk adenoma and colorectal carcinoma. US MSTF recommends shortening the surveillance interval from 10 years to 5 years in patients with low-risk findings on colonoscopy and a first-degree relative with colorectal cancer prior to the age of 60.[14] US MSTF also recommends surveillance with colonoscopy as the preferred method.[14]

3.5. Surveillance colonoscopy in the elderly

There is a significant increase in incidence of both CRC and adenomas with increasing age.[14] The age at which screening colonoscopy should be performed remains controversial. Studies that examined the role of age in surveillance colonoscopy found no association with increasing age and polyp recurrence and concluded it was not necessary to tailor surveillance guidelines by age.[5, 67, 70] Retrospective studies have also shown that comorbidities reduce the benefits of CRC screening. The US MSTF does not give a specific age at which screening can be ceased, but recommends that competing comorbidities and life expectancy should be considered before ordering cancer screening at any age.[14]

3.6. Surveillance colonoscopy and physician nonadherence to guidelines

Nonadherence to guidelines remains a major problem in healthcare policy. The overuse of resources could lead to increased demand for colonoscopy, shifting resources from screening, and thus decreasing the cost-effectiveness of CRC screening program by increasing the unnecessary costs and possibility of adverse events. Alternatively, underuse of colonoscopy in surveillance may lead to suboptimal prevention of colorectal cancer. Schohen, et al. retrospectively evaluated 3,627 screening patients with a history of adenoma removal and found overuse of endoscopy in low-risk patients and underuse in high-risk patients.[71] The reasons for guideline nonadherence include lack of strong evidence to support the surveillance intervals, having multiple guidelines with inconsistent recommendations, lack of awareness of current evidence, fear of legal implication, suboptimal bowel preparation, financial incentive for performing the procedure, and miscommunication between gastroenterologist and primary care providers.[72] Measures to improve adherence to guidelines include continued medical education; written recommendations by endoscopist regarding the follow-up interval after the pathology report; quality improvement interventions such as reminder devices; improvement of bowel preparation quality; automated electronic alerting system[72, 73]; and continuous quality improvement process for colonoscopy (education, monitoring, audits, and financial incentives/penalties).[74]

4. Conclusion

Colorectal cancer screening and surveillance have been shown to provide many benefits. The associated risks are relatively minor and vary greatly on the particular screening test, and surveillance regimen. Patients should be informed that screening and surveillance reduce the risk of colorectal cancer, but may require additional tests and/or procedures to diagnose and manage the pathologic findings. Colorectal cancer screening rate is still suboptimal in the United States and this rate could be improved by dedicated patients and clinician reminders, patients' education, outreach, and follow-up. Screening and surveillance must be targeted to appropriate patients and occur at recommended intervals to ensure proper prevention.

Author details

Rotimi R. Ayoola*, Hamza Abdulla, Evan K. Brady, Muhammed Sherid and Humberto Sifuentes*

*Address all correspondence to: rayoola@gru.edu

Georgia Regents University, Augusta, GA, USA

References

[1] Seigel R, Ward E, Brawley O, Jemal A. Cancer statistics, 2011: the impact of eliminating socioeconomic and racial disparities on premature cancer deaths. *CA Cancer J Clin*. 2011;61:212-36.

[2] Ferlay J, Shin HR, Bray F, Forman D, Mathers C, Parkin DM. Estimates of worldwide burden of cancer in 2008: GLOBOCAN 2008. *Int J Cancer*. 2010;127:2893-2917.

[3] Segnan N, Patnick J, von Karsa L (eds.). *European guidelines for quality assurance in colorectal cancer screening and diagnosis*. 1st edn. Belgium: European Union; 2010. p. 386. DOI: 10.2772/15379

[4] National Cancer Institute. SEER Stat Fact Sheets: Colon and Rectum Cancer [Internet]. 2011. Available from: http://seer.cancer.gov/statfacts/html/colorect.html [Accessed: Feb 2015]

[5] Winawer SJ, Zauber AG, Ho MN, et al. Prevention of colorectal cancer by colonoscopic polypectomy. *N Engl J Med*. 1993;329:1977-81.

[6] Lieberman DA. Screening for colorectal cancer. *N Engl J Med*. 2009;361:1179-87. DOI: 10.1056/NEJMcp0902176

[7] Centers for Disease Control and Prevention (CDC). Vital signs: colorectal cancer screening, incidence, and mortality, 2002-2010. *Morb Mortal Wkly Report*. 2011;60:884.

[8] Winamer S, Fletcher R, Rex D, et al. Colorectal cancer screening and surveillance: clinical guidelines and rationale--update based on new evidence. *Gastroenterology*. 2003;124:544-60.

[9] Baxter NN, Goldwasser MA, PAszat LF, Saskin R, Urbach DR, Rabeneck LA. Association of colonoscopy and death from colorectal cancer. *Ann Int Med*. 2009;150:1-8.

[10] Muller AD, Sonnenberg A. Prevention of colorectal cancer by flexible endoscopy and polypectomy: a case-control study of 32,702 veterans. *Ann Int Med*. 1995;123:904-10.

[11] Singh H, Turner D, Xue L, Targownik LE, Bernstein CN. Risk of developing colorectal cancer following a negative colonoscopy examination: evidence for a 10-year interval between colonoscopies. *JAMA*. 2006;295:2366-73.

[12] Atkin WS, Morson BC, Cuzick J. Long-term risk of colorectal cancer after excision of rectosigmoid adenomas. *N Engl J Med*. 1992;326:658.

[13] Hawk ET, Umar A, Viner JL. Colorectal cancer chemoprevention--an overview of the science. *Gastroenterology*. 2004;126:1423-47.

[14] Preventative Services Task Force. Screening for colorectal cancer: US Preventative Services Task Force recommendation statement. *Ann Int Med*. 2008;149:627-37.

[15] Allison JE, Sakoda LC, Levin TR, et al. Screening for colorectal neoplasms with new fecal occult blood tests: update on performance characteristics. *J Natl Cancer Inst.* 2007;99(19):1462-70.

[16] Mandel JS, Bond JH, Church TR, et al.. Reducing mortality from colorectal cancer by screening for fecal occult blood. *N Engl J Med.* 1993;328:1365-7.

[17] Hardcastle JD, Chamberlain JO, Robinson MH, et al. Randomized controlled trial of faecal-occult blood screening for colorectal cancer. *Lancet.* 1996;348:1472-77.

[18] Kronborg O, Fenger C, Olsen J, Jorgensen OD, Sondergaard O. Randomized study of screening for colorectal cancer with faecal-occult blood test. *Lancet.* 1996;348:1467-71.

[19] Imperiale TF, Wagner DR, Lin CY, Larkin GN, Rogge JD, Ransohoff DF. Risk of advanced proximal neoplasms in asymptomatic adults according to the distal colorectal findings. *N Engl J Med.* 2000;343:169-74.

[20] Ahlquist DA, Sargent DJ, Loprinzi CL, et al. Stool DNA and occult blood testing for screen detection of colorectal neoplasia. *Ann Int Med.* 2008;149:441-50.

[21] Levin B, Lieberman DA, McFarland B, et al. Screening and surveillance for early detection of colorectal cancer and adenomatous polyps, 2008: a joint guideline from the American Cancer Society, the US Multi-Society Task Force on Colorectal Cancer, and the American College of Radiology. *Gastroenterology.* 2008;134:1570-95.

[22] Whitlock EP, Lin JS, Liles E, Beil TL, Fu R. Screening for colorectal cancer: a targeted, updated systematic review for US Preventative Task Force. *Ann Int Med.* 2008;149:638-65.

[23] Itzkowitz SH, Jandorf L, Brand R, et al. Improved fecal DNA test for colorectal cancer screening. *Clin Gastroenterol Hepatol.* 2007;5:111-7.

[24] Johnson CD, Chem MH, Toledano AY, et al. Accuracy of CT colonography for detection of large adenomas and cancers. *N Engl J Med.* 2008;359:1207-1

[25] Shelby JV, Friedman GD, Quesenberry CP Jr, Weiss NS. A case-control study of screening sigmoidoscopy and mortality from colorectal cancer. *N Engl J Med.* 1992;326:653-7.

[26] Schoenfeld P, Cash B, Flood A, et al. Colonoscopic screening of average-risk women for colorectal cancer. *N Engl J Med.* 2005;352:2061-8.

[27] Lieberman DA, Holub JL, Moravec MD, Eisen GM, Peters D, Morris CD. Prevalence of colon polyps detected by colonoscopy screening in asymptomatic black and white patients. *JAMA.* 2008;300:1417-22.

[28] Pickhardt PJ, Choi R, Hwang I, et al. Computed tomographic virtual colonoscopy to screen for colorectal neoplasia in asymptomatic adults. *N Engl J Med.* 2003;349:2191-200.

[29] Cotton PB, Durkalski VL, Pineau BC, et al. Computed tomography (virtual colonoscopy): a multicenter comparison with standard colonoscopy for detection of colorectal neoplasia. *JAMA*. 2004;291:1713-9.

[30] Rockey DC, Paulson E, Neidzwiecki D, et al. Analysis of air contrast barium enema, computer tomographic colonography and colonoscopy: prospective comparison. *Lancet*. 2005;365:305-11.

[31] Pignone M, Saha S, Hoerger T, Mandelblatt J. Cost-effectiveness analyses of colorectal cancer screening: a systematic review for US Preventive Services Task Force. *Ann Int Med*. 2001;137(2):96-104.

[32] Lasa JS, Moore R, Peralta AD, Dima G, Zubiaurre I, Arguello M, et al. Impact of the endoscopic teaching process on colonic adenoma detection. *Revista de Gastroenterol de Mexico* (Engl Ed). 2014;79:155-8.

[33] Hol L, Wilschut JA, van Ballegooijen M, et al. Screening for colorectal cancer: random comparison of guaiac and immunochemical faecal occult blood testing at different cut-off levels. *Br J Cancer*. 2009;100:1103-10.

[34] Parra-Blanco A, Gimeno-Garcia AZ, Quintero E, et al. Diagnostic accuracy of immunochemical versus guaiac faecal occult blood tests for colorectal screening. *J Gastroenterol*. 2010;45:703-12.

[35] Van Rossum LG, van Rijn AF, Laheij RJ, et al. Random comparison of guaiac and immunochemical fecal occult blood tests for colorectal cancer in screening population. *Gastroenterology*. 2008;135:82-90.

[36] Levi Z, Birkenfeld S, Vilkin A, et al. A higher detection rate for colorectal cancer and advanced adenomatous polyp for screening with immunochemical fecal occult blood test than guaiac fecal occult blood test, despite lower compliance rate: a prospective, controlled, feasibility study. *Int J Cancer*. 2011;128:2415-24.

[37] Quintero E, Castells A, Bujanda L, Cubiella J, Salas D, Lanas A, et al. Colonoscopy versus fecal immunochemical testing in colorectal cancer screening. *N Engl J Med*. 2012;366(8):697-706. DOI: 10.1056/NEJMoa1108895

[38] Yang DX, Gross CP, Soulos PR, Yu JB. Estimating the magnitude of colorectal cancers prevented during the era of screening. *Cancer*. 2014;120(18):2893-901.

[39] Wolf WI, Shinya H. Polypectomy via the fiberoptic colonoscope: removal of neoplasms beyond the reach of the sigmoidoscope. *N Engl J Med*. 1973;288:329-32.

[40] Winawer SJ, Stewart ET, Zauber AG, et al. A comparison of colonoscopy and double-contrast barium enema for surveillance after polypectomy. *N Engl J Med*. 2000; 342:1766-72

[41] Toma J, Paszat LF, Gunraj N, Rabeneck L. Rates of new or missed colorectal cancer after barium enema and their risk factors: a population-based study. *Am J Gastroenterol.* 2008;103:3142.

[42] Centers for Disease Control and Prevention (CDC). Vital signs: colorectal cancer screening test use – United States, 2012. *Morb Mortal Wkly Rep.* 2013;62:881.

[43] Weissfeld JL, Schoen RE, Pinsky PF, et al. Flexible sigmoidoscopy in the PLCO cancer screening trial: results from the baseline screening examination of a randomized trial. *J Natl Cancer Inst.* 2005;97:989-97.

[44] Atkin WS, Edwards R, Kralj-Hans I, et al. Once-only flexible sigmoidoscopy screening in prevention of colorectal cancer: a multicentre randomized controlled trial. *Lancet.* 2010;375:1324-33.

[45] Schoen RE, Pinsky PF, Weissfeld JL. Colorectal-Cancer Incidence and Mortality with screening Flexible Sigmoidoscopy. *N Engl J Med.* 2012: 366:2345-2357

[46] Waye JD, Aisenberg J, Rubin PH. Indications and contraindications for colonscopy. In: *Practical Colonscopy.* Oxford, UK: Blackwell Publishing; 2013. p. 24-9. DOI: 10.1002/9781118553442

[47] Wang YR, Cangemi JR, Loftus EV, Picco MF. Risk of colorectal cancer after colonoscopy compared with flexible sigmoidoscopy or no lower endoscopy among older patients in the United States, 1998-2005. *Mayo Clinic Proc.* 2013;88:464-70.

[48] Evans WK, Wolfson MC, Flanagan WM, Shin J, Goffin J, Miller AB, et al. Canadian cancer risk management model: evaluation of cancer control. *Int J Tech Assess Health Care.* 2013;29:131-9.

[49] Jemal A, Seigel R, Ward E, Hao Y, Xu J, Thun MC. Cancer statistics, 2009. *CA Cancer J Clin.* 2009;59:225-249.

[50] Cairns SR, Scholefield JH, et al. Guidelines for colorectal cancer screening and surveillance in moderate and high risk groups (update from 2002). *Gut.* 2010; 59:666-690.

[51] Baron TH, Smyrk TC, Rex DK. Recommended intervals between screening and surveillance colonoscopies. *Mayo Clin Proc.* 2013;88(8):854-8. DOI: 10.1016/j.mayocp.2013.04.023

[52] Waye J, Braunfeld S. Surveillance intervals after colonoscopic polypectomy. *Endoscopy.* 1982;14(3):79-81.

[53] Winawer S, Zauber A, O'Brien M, et al. Randomized comparison of surveillance intervals after colonoscopic removal of newly diagnosed adenomatous polyps. *N Engl J Med.* 1993;328:901-6.

[54] Atkin W, Williams C, Macrae F, et al. Randomized study of surveillance intervals after removal of colorectal adenomas at colonoscopy. *Gut.* 1992;33:S52.

[55] Neugut A, Jacobson J, Ashan H, et al. Incidence and recurrence rates of colorectal adenomas--a prospective study. *Gastroenterology*. 1995;108:402-8.

[56] Atkin WS, Saunders BP. Surveillance guidelines after removal of colorectal adenomatous polyps. *Gut*. 2002;51 (Suppl. V):v6-vv9.

[57] Nishihara R, Wu K, Lochhead P, Morikawa T, Liao X, Qian ZR, et al. Long-term colorectal cancer incidence and mortality after lower endoscopy. *N Engl J Med*. 2013;369(12):1095-105. DOI: 10.1056/NEJMoa1301969

[58] Saini SD, Schoenfeld P, Vijan S. Surveillance colonoscopy is cost-effective for patients with adenomas who are at high risk of colorectal cancer. *Gastroenterology*. 2010;138(7): 2292-9. DOI: 10.1053/j.gastro.2010.03.004

[59] Murphy CC, Lewis CL, Golin CE, Sandler RS. Underuse of surveillance colonoscopy in patients at increased risk of colorectal cancer. *Am J Gastroenterol*. Forthcoming. DOI: 10.1038/ajg.2014.344

[60] Martinex ME, Ahnen D, Greenberg ER. One-year risk for advanced colorectal neoplasia. *Ann Int Med*. 2013;158(8):639. DOI: 10.7326/0003-4819-158-8-201304160-00019

[61] Rex DK, Ahnen DJ, Baron JA, Batts KP, Burke CA, Burt RW, et al. Serrated lesions of the colorectum: review and recommendations from an expert panel. *Am J Gastroenterol*. 2012;107:1315-29. DOI: 10.1038/ajg.2012.161

[62] Tinmouth J, Henry P, Hsieh E, Baxter NN, Hilsden RJ, Elizabeth McGregor S, et al. Sessile serrate polyps at screening colonoscopy: have they been underdiagnosed? *Am J Gastroenterol*. 2014;109(11):1698-704. DOI: 10.1038/ajg.2014.78

[63] Pohl H, Srivastava A, Bensen SP, Anderson P, Rothstein RI, Gordon SR, et al. Incomplete polyp resection during colonscopy--results of the complete adenoma resection (CARE) study. *Gastroenterology*. 2013;144(1):74-80. DOI: 10.1053/j.gastro.2012.09.043

[64] Hassan C, Quientero E, Dumonceau JM, Regula J, Brandao C, Chaussade S, et al. Post-polypectomy colonoscopy surveillance: European Society of Gastroenterology Endoscopy (ESGE) guideline. *Endoscopy*. 2013;45:842-51. DOI: 10.1055/s-0033-1344548

[65] Bosman FT, Carniero F, Hruban Rh, Theise ND (eds.). WHO classification of tumours of digestive system. 4th edn. Geneva, Switzerland: WHO/IARC Press; 2010. p. 417.

[66] Kaminski MF, Hassan C, Bisschops R, Pohl J, Pellise M, Dekker E, et al. Advanced imaging for detection and differentiation of colorectal neoplasia: European Society of Gastroenterology Endoscopy (ESGE) guideline. *Endoscopy*. 2014;46:435-49. DOI: 10.1055/s-0034-1365348

[67] Day LW, Walter LC, Velayos F. Colorectal cancer screening and surveillance in the elderly patient. *Am J Gastroenterol*. 2011;106(7):1197-206. DOI: 10.1038/ajg.2011.128

[68] Noshirwani KC, van Stolk RU, Rybicki LA, et al. Adenoma size and number are predictive of adenoma recurrence: implications for surveillance colonoscopy. *Gastrointest Endosc*. 2000;51(4):433-7.

[69] Harewood GC, Lawlor GO. Incident rates of colonic neoplasia according to age and gender: implications for surveillance colonoscopy intervals. *J Clin Gastroenterol*. 2005;39(10):894-9.

[70] Harewood GC, Lawlor GO, Larson MV. Incident rates of colonic neoplasia in older patients: when should we stop screening? *J Gastroenterol Hepatol*. 2006;21(6):1021-5.

[71] Schoen RE, Pinsky FP, Weissfeld JL, Yokochi LA, Reding DJ, Hayes RB, et al. Utilization of surveillance colonoscopy in community practice. *Gastroenterology*. 2010;138(1): 73-81. DOI: 10.1053/j.gastro.2009.09.062

[72] Sarfaty M, Wender R. How to increase colorectal cancer screening rates in practice. *CA Cancer J Clin*. 2007;57(6):354-66.

[73] Leffler DA, Neeman N, Rabb JM, Shin JY, Landon BE, Pallav K, et al. An alerting system improves adherence to follow-up recommendations for colonoscopic examinations. *Gastroenterology*. 2011;140:1166-73. DOI: 10.1053/j.gastro.2011.01.003

[74] Rex DK, Petrini JL, Baron TH, Chak A, Cohen J, Deal SE, et al. Quality indicators for colonoscopy. Am J Gastroenterol. 2006;101(4):873-85.

Section 2

Indications and Outcomes

Chapter 3

Colonoscopy — Indications and Contraindications

Jigar Bhagatwala, Arpit Singhal, Summer Aldrugh,
Muhammed Sherid, Humberto Sifuentes and
Subbaramiah Sridhar

Additional information is available at the end of the chapter

http://dx.doi.org/10.5772/61097

Abstract

This chapter discusses some of the major indications and contraindications for colonoscopy. Advances in colonoscopic techniques have expanded the role of colonoscopy beyond conventional screening, surveillance, and diagnosis to various complex therapeutic and interventional utilities. Several guidelines with new information are being published and updated regularly in the field of colonoscopy and are currently used in clinical practice. However, there is still a lack of well-designed randomized clinical trials investigating the role of colonoscopy in early diagnosis and treatment of various conditions and its impact on long-term survival and disease status. Nevertheless, retrospective observational studies and a few randomized clinical trials abundantly supply data supporting the role of colonoscopy in the diagnosis and management of colonic pathologies in the absence of comparable alternatives.

Keywords: Colonoscopy, Indication, Contraindication, Screening, Surveillance, Diagnostic, Therapeutic

1. Introduction

In the 1960s, Drs. William Wolff and Hiromi Shinya developed a way to probe the full length of the colon using a tube with electronic sensors [1]. Since its inception, colonoscopy has become a very popular method for screening of colorectal cancers and for treating a variety of conditions of the lower gastrointestinal tract. The decision to perform colonoscopy should take into account the indication and contraindication for the procedure, the risks of the procedure, and the cost. A key quality measure of colonoscopy is the indication for the procedure, because as high as 20-50% of colonoscopies are performed for inappropriate indications [2]. Performing colonoscopy for inappropriate indications not only exposes patients to procedure-related complications such as bowel perforation, bleeding, infection, and cardiovascular events, but also increases on the health-care-related cost. Therefore, several societies including the American Society of Gastrointestinal Endoscopy (ASGE) and the European Panel on the Appropriateness of Gastrointestinal Endoscopy (EPAGE), have established guidelines for appropriate use of colonoscopy. In this chapter, we aim to outline the common indications and contraindications for performing colonoscopy and detail the evidence supporting the facts.

2. Indications for colonoscopy (table 1)

2.1. Lower gastrointestinal (GI) bleeding

Lower GI bleeding may occur in the form of occult bleeding, melena, scant intermittent hematochezia, or severe hematochezia [3]. Lower GI bleeding from any cause requires colonoscopy either urgently or routinely. Patients with occult GI bleeding require colonoscopy to exclude malignant or adenomatous etiologies. Patients who are not good candidates for colonoscopy can be evaluated using CT colonography [4]. In patients presenting with melena, upper GI endoscopy is performed first to identify any upper GI causes. If the upper GI endoscopy does not reveal a source of bleeding, colonoscopy is then indicated to identify any colonic source. Intermittent scant hematochezia can be diagnosed by anoscopy with/without sigmoidoscopy for low-lying lesions in the anus, rectum, and sigmoid in patients who are younger than 40. However, colonoscopy may still be required if a definitive source cannot be identified. On the other hand, colonoscopy is the recommended procedure for patients with intermittent hematochezia who have one of the following risk factors: age >50, family history of colon cancer, or other alarming symptoms such as weight loss, anemia, and change in bowel habits [5, 6]. Overall, colonoscopy has been reported to have a higher yield than other modalities such as proctosigmoidoscopy, single-contrast barium studies, or combined flexible sigmoidoscopy and double-contrast barium enema for diagnosis of lower GI bleeding. In case of severe hematochezia, hemodynamic stability determines the diagnostic and therapeutic approach [7-9]. In hemodynamically stable patients, urgent (within 8-24 h) colonoscopy is recommended [10-13]. In critically ill patients, upper endoscopy is indicated first followed by colonoscopy after excluding the upper GI tract as the source of bleeding [14]. The therapeutic indications of colonoscopy for the treatment of lower GI bleeding are discussed separately in this chapter.

http://dx.doi.org/10.5772/61097

Indications for colonoscopy:
1.Lower GI bleeding
2.Screening and surveillance of colorectal polyps and cancers: a. Colon cancer b. Surveillance after polypectomy c. Colorectal cancer post-resection surveillance d. Inflammatory bowel diseases
3.Acute and chronic diarrhea
4.Therapeutic indications for colonoscopy: a. Excision and ablation of lesions b. Treatment of lower GI bleeding c. Colonic decompression d. Dilation of colonic stenosis e. Foreign body removal
5.Miscellaneous indications: a. Abnormal radiological examinations b. Isolated unexplained abdominal pain c. Chronic constipation d. Preoperative and intraoperative localization of colonic lesions

Table 1. Indications for colonoscopy

2.2. Screening and surveillance of colorectal polyps and cancers

2.2.1. Colon cancer

According to the World Health Organization report in 2012, colorectal cancer (CRC) is the third most common cancer in men (746,000 cases, 10% of the total) and the second in women (614,000 cases, 9.2% of the total) worldwide. In 2014, the American Cancer Society predicted that about 136,830 people would be diagnosed with colorectal cancer in the United States, and about 50,310 people were predicted to die of the disease. Recent studies show declining in the CRC incidence and mortality rates, which have been attributed to the awareness of the risk factors and reduced exposure to them, the effect of early detection and prevention through polypectomy, and improved treatment [15]. The recommendations for screening colonoscopies are divided based on the known risk factor profile: 1) screening in the average-risk population and 2) screening in patients with a family history of colon cancer.

In the average-risk patient, current American, European, and Asian guidelines recommend beginning CRC screening with colonoscopy at the age of 50 years and every 10 years thereafter regardless of the gender. However, the American College of Gastroenterology recommends that the screening colonoscopy begin at the age of 45 years in African Americans [16, 17]. Published evidence favoring the effectiveness of colonoscopy in reducing mortality from CRC by routine colonoscopy is insufficient because of a lack of randomized controlled trials and the limited consensus in guidelines on the appropriateness of colonoscopy. However, a few studies have modeled and predicted the impact of screening colonoscopy on CRC incidence and mortality using various transition models in hypothetical average-risk individuals aged 50 years. These studies have found that initial screening colonoscopy and repeat colonoscopy every 10 years might reduce CRC incidence by 58% and the reduction in CRC mortality is approximately 64% [18, 19]. In the average-risk individuals, yearly fecal occult blood testing (FOBT) and flexible sigmoidoscopy (FSIG) every 3 years are also accepted methods of screening for CRC. A follow-up colonoscopy, however, is warranted to completely visualize the entire length of the colon for patients with positive FOBT results or FSIG findings of adenoma in the distal colon [20-23].

Family history of CRC is a major risk factor for CRC. It has been estimated that the first-degree relatives of CRC patients have two- to threefold increased risk of dying from CRC, and the risk is inversely associated with the age of diagnosis of the affected family member [24]. Patients with a single first-degree relative with CRC or advanced adenoma (adenoma ≥1 cm in size, with high-grade dysplasia, or villous elements) diagnosed at age ≥60 years are recommended to undergo routine CRC screening same as an average-risk individual beginning at age 50 years. On the other hand, patients with a single first-degree relative with CRC or advanced adenoma diagnosed at age <60 years, or two first-degree relatives with CRC or advanced adenomas should receive colonoscopy every 5 years beginning at age 40, or 10 years earlier than the age at diagnosis of the youngest affected relative, whichever comes first [16]. The data supporting these recommendations emerge from the retrospective studies rather than the randomized control trials [25, 26].

Patients with a family history of hereditary nonpolyposis colorectal cancer (HNPCC), an autosomal dominant disease, are recommended to start the CRC screening at the age of 20-25 years or 10 years prior to the earliest age of HNPCC diagnosis in the patient's family member, whichever comes first. The recommended interval for colonoscopy is every 1-2 years until age 40, then annually thereafter [27-30]. This condition, in particular, has two-thirds of adenomas occurring on the right side and warrants colonoscopy for complete colonic surveillance [31]. Indications for performing colonoscopy in individuals with a history of familial adenomatous polyposis (FAP) are guideline-dependent after genetic testing returns positive. FSIG and colonoscopy have not been compared head-to-head regarding their effectiveness and reducing mortality in patients with FAP in the clinical trials and, as such, either FSIG or colonoscopy annually is recommended, starting at the age of 10-12 years [16]. A colonoscopy is deemed necessary when polyps are detected on FSIG and a decision to perform polypectomy is made.

2.2.2. Surveillance after polypectomy

Post-polypectomy surveillance constitutes 20% of the performed colonoscopies, thereby constituting a large share in the amount of health care expenditure [32, 33]. Adhering to the indications for the repeat colonoscopy for the surveillance of CRC after the first colonoscopy, therefore, is very important as earlier colonoscopy can increase the risks to the patient and add to the health care cost whereas delaying the surveillance can also increase the risks by increasing the chances of missed interval cancers. Various observational studies report a 2-5%

risk of an advanced neoplasia 5-10 years after a negative colonoscopy, a risk that is comparable to the risk of advanced colonic neoplasia in the average-risk patients undergoing their first colonoscopy [34-39]. Moreover, the risk of developing CRC 10 years after a negative colonoscopy is reported to be significantly lower (adjusted OR 0.26) [36, 40], supporting the current recommendation of repeat colonoscopy every 10 years in the average-risk general population.

Although the detection and removal of polyp(s) can offer a significant reduction in the mortality of CRC, the development of interval cancers, i.e., the cancers occurring after the initial colonoscopy with polypectomy, appears to be the highest in the first 3-5 years. In 2012, the United States Multi-Society Task Force (USMSTF) published a revision of the 2006 guidelines on post-polypectomy surveillance and divided recommendations based on the presence of polyp(s) (hyperplastic vs. adenomatous), the number and the size of adenomatous polyp(s), villous component and high-grade dysplasia in the polyp, and the presence of serrated lesions or serrated polyposis syndrome (>20 serrated polyps of any size throughout the colon) at baseline colonoscopy. In 2013, the European Society of Gastrointestinal Endoscopy (ESGE) published its post-polypectomy surveillance guidelines, stratifying risk into: low risk (1-2 adenomas <1 cm), intermediate risk (3-4 small adenomas or one >1 cm), and high risk (>5 small adenomas or >3 adenomas with at least one >1 cm) based on the first colonoscopy. According to the USMSTF guideline, it is indicated that patients with 1-2 tubular adenomas <1 cm have a repeat colonoscopy in 10 years; whereas patients with a high-risk adenoma (defined as adenoma with villous histology, high-grade dysplasia, adenoma>10 mm, or three or more adenomas) are recommended to have surveillance interval of 3 years. According to the ESGE guideline, the high-risk group should undergo surveillance at 1 year, the intermediate-risk group at 3-yearly intervals until two consecutive examinations are negative, and the low-risk group requires no surveillance colonoscopy or 5-yearly colonoscopy until one negative examination after which surveillance can be discontinued. The evidence supporting the indications in the arena of surveillance for the serrated polyp is insufficient. According to the USMSTF guideline, sessile serrated polyp(s) <1 cm with no dysplasia should be considered low risk and can be followed at a 5-year interval. However, sessile serrated polyp(s) ≥1 cm or sessile serrated polyp with dysplasia or serrated adenoma should undergo surveillance at 3 years and serrated polyposis syndrome should be surveyed annually. The ESGE recommends that patients with serrated polyps <10 mm in size without dysplasia should be classified as low risk, whereas patients with large serrated polyps (≥10 mm) or those with dysplasia as high risk and undergo surveillance accordingly. Patients with ≥5 serrated polyps proximal to the sigmoid, of which ≥2 are sized ≥10mm, or with ≥20 serrated polyps of any size are classified as serrated polyposis and should be referred for genetic testing.

2.2.3. CRC post-resection surveillance

There are no clear survival benefits for performing colonoscopy in patients who have had colon cancer resection. However, a majority of the groups and societies such as American Cancer Society (ACS), and a joint American Cancer Society/US Multi-Society Task Force on Colorectal Cancer, Cancer Care Ontario [41-44], recommend post CRC resection surveillance. An indication to perform colonoscopy in these patients will help detect metachronous CRCs and polyps as well as anastomotic recurrences of the initial primary cancer at a stage that would allow further treatment. Currently, a follow-up colonoscopy is indicated at 1 year after the surgical removal of CRC. If no new cancer or polyp(s) is identified, a colonoscopy is repeated at 3 years and at 5 years if the findings are negative for interval development of cancer. An exception to this indication is HNPCC, which requires colonoscopic surveillance every 1-2 years regardless of the surgical resection of the cancer.

2.2.4. *Inflammatory bowel diseases and other colitis*

The indications for colonoscopy in inflammatory bowel disease (IBD), namely ulcerative colitis (UC) and Crohn's disease (CD) fall under a large spectrum. Colonoscopic diagnosis and differentiation between the UC and CD, assessment of the extent and severity of disease activity, treatment effectiveness, surveillance of malignancies, and endoscopic treatment, such as stricture dilation, are all within the scope of colonoscopy and its indications in IBD. Currently, American, European, and other international societies and guideline-defining bodies recommend endoscopic visualization of the entire colon for the initial diagnosis of IBD and other colitis [45-48]. The clinical presentation and laboratory data characterizing both diseases may overlap but endoscopic visualization of the mucosa of the rectum, colon, and terminal ileum, and the extent of the disease involvement may help differentiate the disease processes. Moreover, colonoscopy offers the opportunity to perform biopsy, which is the major advantage of colonoscopy. Unless contraindicated because of severe colitis or possible toxic megacolon, a full colonoscopy with intubation of the terminal ileum should be performed during the initial evaluation of patients with a clinical presentation suggestive of IBD. Ileoscopy is superior for the diagnosis of CD of the terminal ileum when compared with radiological methods, especially for mild lesions [49, 50]. During the colonoscopic examination, biopsy samples should be obtained both from areas affected by the disease and from unaffected areas. After initiating therapy, a smaller number of biopsy samples may be necessary to confirm the diagnosis. In postsurgical follow-up, biopsies of the neoterminal ileum are indicated when disease recurrence is suspected. In patients who have undergone ileal pouch-anal anastomosis, biopsies of the afferent limb are indicated when Crohn's disease is suspected [46]. Other forms of colitis, such as drug-induced, infectious, vascular, and radiation colitis also present in a similar pattern and require colonoscopy at baseline for the diagnosis and the assessment of severity.

Patients with IBD have an increased risk of CRC compared to those without IBD [51-55]. In fact, CRC accounts for one-sixth of ulcerative colitis-related deaths [56]. There is a lack of randomized control studies demonstrating the effectiveness of colonoscopy in improving survival in the IBD patients from CRC. However, numerous observational studies have reported that colonoscopic surveillance of CRC in IBD offers early detection of cancers and improves CRC-related survival in IBD patients [57, 58]. In a retrospective study of 6,823 patients with IBD in US tertiary referral hospitals followed-up for at least 3 years, the incidence of CRC among patients without a recent colonoscopy was 2.7% which was significantly higher than among patients with a recent colonoscopy (1.6%) [59]. Additionally, a colonoscopy within 6-36 months before diagnosis was associated with a 64% reduction in mortality rate [59].

According to most guidelines, colonoscopies are indicated for CRC screening starting at 8-10 years from initiation of IBD-related symptoms [48, 53, 60-62]. The National Institute for Health and Clinical Excellence (NICE) London 2011 guideline, however, recommends only offering colonoscopic surveillance to patients with Crohn's colitis involving more than 1 segment of the colon or left-sided or more extensive UC, but not isolated ulcerative proctitis. Most guidelines recommend yearly follow-up colonoscopy for high-risk patients (those with primary sclerosing cholangitis, extensive colitis, active endoscopic or histologic inflammation, a family history of CRC in a first-degree relative before 50 years of age, personal history of dysplasia, presence of strictures on colonoscopy, and, possibly, gender), and every 2-5 years for those without major risk factors.

2.3. Acute and chronic diarrhea

Patients presenting with acute diarrhea should undergo initial evaluation with stool studies. If blood and stool cultures are inconclusive, or if symptoms persist or worsen despite empiric therapy, then colonoscopy is indicated due to its high diagnostic yield [63]. For most patients with chronic diarrhea, patients with suspected acute diffuse *Clostridium Difficile* colitis, pregnant patients, patients with predominantly left-sided symptoms (tenesmus/urgency) and patients with multiple morbidities, a flexible sigmoidoscopy can be used for the initial evaluation. Even if patients have macroscopically normal-appearing mucosa, biopsies must be obtained to exclude microscopic diseases. If flexible sigmoidoscopy yields inconclusive results, if diarrhea persists, or if there is suspicion of inflammatory bowel disease (IBD) or cancer, then colonoscopy should be the next investigative study.

Histology is an integral component of colonoscopic evaluation of chronic diarrhea because several diseases, such as microscopic colitis, eosinophilic colitis, amyloidosis, and IBD, may appear normal on endoscopy but are abnormal on microscopy. In patients undergoing colonoscopy for chronic diarrhea, IBD or colitis is the most likely disease to be detected [64]. Microscopic colitis can be lymphocytic or collagenous and is characterized by nonbloody, watery diarrhea. On endoscopy, microscopic colitis can be missed because of patchy colonic involvement. Even if mucosa appears normal endoscopically, multiple biopsies from both sides of the colon are necessary to avoid missing microscopic colitis [65]. If there is suspicion of inflammatory diarrhea, then a biopsy of the terminal ileum is helpful in the diagnosis. However, a biopsy of the terminal ileum has the highest diagnostic yield in patients with known or suspected Crohn's disease, terminal ileal abnormalities on imaging, or endoscopic findings of ulcers, ileitis, or erosions [66].

Colonoscopy is not routinely used to evaluate acute diarrhea because it is commonly due to infectious etiology. If stool tests are negative and/or if diarrhea persists, then endoscopy is indicated. An additional important exception is the case of an immunocompromised patient. In a patient with diarrhea with HIV, organ or bone marrow transplant, or on immunosuppressive medications, a colonoscopy with biopsy is necessary to exclude CMV colitis and graft versus host disease (GVHD). In such cases, colonoscopic evaluation of diarrhea has higher sensitivity and cost-effectiveness than FSIG [67]. Patients who undergo stem cell transplant often present with diarrhea in the initial 3 months following transplantation. In these patients, abnormal mucosa on endoscopy has not been shown to correlate with biopsy results. Therefore, biopsies of normal and abnormal-appearing mucosa are indicated, especially of the distal colon, which has the highest diagnostic yield in patients undergoing endoscopy for gastrointestinal symptoms [68]. Based on the location of highest diagnostic yield, a flexible sigmoidoscopy with distal colon biopsy is indicated in patients with diarrhea suspected of acute GVHD. However, some centers endorse combined upper GI endoscopy as well as colonoscopy in patients following hematopoietic stem cell transplantation to diagnose disease more quickly.

2.4. Therapeutic indications for colonoscopy

2.4.1. Excision and ablation of lesions

Endoscopic mucosal resection (EMR) is a method for treating early CRC. Most adenomas and intramucosal cancers can be removed by EMR. For tumors larger than 2 cm, EMR is less likely to achieve complete resection (histopathologically tumor-free lateral and vertical margins of the resected specimens) [69, 70]. Another method, known as endoscopic submucosal dissection (ESD) is also performed in several countries. The procedure is simpler than the laparoscopic colectomy but is time-consuming and carries a higher risk of perforation than EMR. ESD is indicated in lesions >2 cm, lesions that are suspected to be invasive submucosal cancer, and mucosal lesions with fibrosis or local residual early cancer after endoscopic resection. The rate of complete resection for large colorectal tumors by ESD has been reported to be 80-98.9% [71-74]. However, both procedures are operator-dependent and have limited data supporting their use.

2.4.2. Treatment of lower GI bleeding

Treatment of acute lower GI bleeding from any sources described earlier is indicated either urgently or as an elective procedure. In case of urgent colonoscopy, the colon is prepared using polyethylene glycol based solution administered orally or via nasogastric tube. Currently, metallic clip placement, thermal coagulation, and epinephrine injection are the available methods. Depending on the lesion and the severity of bleeding, colonoscopic intervention with any one of these methods is indicated as the first step in achieving hemostasis. In case of persistent diverticular bleeding, a bleeding vessel can be treated with metallic clip placement [75, 76]. Vascular ectasias can be treated with either thermal or epinephrine injection, though thermal cauterization has 87% of success rate [77]. Cases where a definite bleeding site cannot be located or cases where the visualization of the bleeding source is poor due to inadequate views due to bleeding need referral for angiographic or surgical treatment.

2.4.3. Colonic decompression

Acute colonic obstruction is a common presentation of colon cancer and, often, the presenting patient is in poor overall health making surgical intervention a suboptimal choice. Since 1990, the utility of colonoscopic interventions via either self-expanding metal stent (SEMS), placement of a decompression tube, or tumor debulking has become very popular and has been studied more frequently in recent years in various populations. Endoscopic interventions serve as a bridge to surgery or as a palliative measure in patients who are poor surgical candidates. A majority of the studies comparing SEMS placement with surgery has reported high clinical success rates (92%), better symptomatic relief, lower complication rates (<5%), cost-effectiveness, and higher patient acceptance and shorter hospital stay with endoscopic SEMS placement [78-83]. Argon plasma coagulation (APC) and snare polypectomy have been used to treat colonic obstruction and maintain luminal patency, and are good alternatives to endoscopic SEMS in treating colonic obstruction [84-86].

Endoscopic decompression of an acute colonic pseudo-obstruction or Ogilvie syndrome is another therapeutic indication for colonoscopy. The etiology of this condition is multifactorial (post-intraabdominal surgery, sepsis, hypothyroidism, neurological disorder, spinal cord injury, etc.) in the absence of a true mechanical obstruction. Bowel ischemia and perforation are dreaded complications and management is often conservative, involving the correction of the underlying disorder. However, in cases where the initial management fails, colonoscopic decompression is indicated [87, 88].

Colonoscopy is also used for decompression of sigmoid and cecal volvulus. Volvulus is a condition in which a part of colon twists upon itself. Due to venous congestion and obstruction to blood flow, tissue viability becomes a major issue. Patients presenting with signs of perforation, peritonitis, bowel necrosis or profound hemodynamic instability need immediate surgery. However, patients with less severe sigmoid and cecal volvulus can be managed endoscopically [89, 90]. Endoscopic correction of sigmoid volvulus achieves better success rates than the correction of cecal volvulus and is associated with a lesser need for surgical intervention [91]. A study by Oren and colleagues reported that sigmoidoscopic correction of sigmoid volvulus with a rectal tube was successful in 78% of patients [92]. Nevertheless, the rate of recurrence of sigmoid volvulus is high, ultimately requiring surgical treatment [93]. Cecal volvulus has been treated endoscopically but due to the high failure rate, often requires surgical intervention for most patients. Surgeons usually combine operative detorsion of cecal volvulus with right hemicolectomy (to prevent recurrence) and either a primary anastomosis or an ileostomy with mucus fistula. In medically unstable, high-risk patients who are poor surgical candidates or have poor vascular supplies to the cecum, cecal volvulus detorsion may be achieved with a cecostomy and cecopexy, which also are associated with significant morbidity and mortality [94]. Colonic volvuluses in other areas such as flexural territories are less common and the indication to perform colonoscopic interventions in these situations is not well studied.

2.4.4. Dilation of colonic stenosis

Colonoscopic intervention of stenotic lesions such as anastomotic strictures and strictures caused by IBD are among the common indications for performing colonoscopy. Several studies have reported high success rate with a low complications rate. However, recurrence is common. The methods commonly employed for the treatment of colonic stenosis are balloon dilation with or without steroid injection and electro-incision, all of which have been shown to have a variable amount of success [95-101].

2.4.5. Foreign body removal

The current management of the foreign bodies lying in the lower GI tract is based on the type of foreign body, the proximity to the anus, the injury to the adjacent structure, as well as the surgical and endoscopic expertise at the health care center. A foreign body in the GI tract presents after voluntary or involuntary insertion or ingestion of the foreign body. Very often, the patient tries to manipulate the object and attempts self-exploration to remove it before presenting to the hospital. Endoscopy provides an opportunity to avoid abdominal exploration. However if the radiological exam or clinical presentation indicates perforation or higher-lying object(s), colonoscopy may fail and may pose a delay in surgical management [102-106].

2.5. Miscellaneous indications

2.5.1. Abnormal radiological examination

Colonoscopy is commonly performed after an abnormal or suspicious radiological finding in the search for true pathological lesions such as cancers or ulcerative lesions. Filling defect or mucosal defect on barium enema or a luminal narrowing on barium enema or CT scan is routinely evaluated with a colonoscopy. Patients presenting with symptoms suggestive of acute diverticulitis with supportive CT scan findings also need to be evaluated with colonoscopy, but only after the acute inflammation has resolved. Air insufflation during colonoscopy in acute diverticulitis can lead to the bowel perforation and is considered a contraindication. A luminal defect or polyp(s) on CT scan or CT colonography is usually followed-up by a colonoscopy when feasible. However, controversy exists between the American College of Radiology, the American Gastroenterology Association, and American College of Gastroenterology regarding the size and number of polyps on CT colonography that meet the requirement for colonoscopy [107-109]. Patients with abnormal positron emission tomography (PET) scan showing a possible colorectal lesion should undergo colonoscopic evaluation. Nevertheless, in the light of insufficient clinical data, the indications for colonoscopy after abnormal radiological exam are based on individual presentation, availability of the endoscopist, age, and other comorbidities of the patient.

2.5.2. Isolated unexplained abdominal pain

Patients presenting with symptoms of chronic (>3 months) abdominal pain and nonspecific abdominal discomfort might require colonoscopy. In the era of thorough radiologic studies, the need for colonoscopy emerges after noninvasive diagnostic modalities fail and symptoms persist. There is no clear indication for performing colonoscopy in patients presenting with unexplained abdominal pain or discomfort. A detailed history and physical examination provide diagnostic clues but a diagnostic workup often ends up requiring colonoscopy. The diagnostic yield of colonoscopy has been previously studied in retrospective studies. For example, in a study by Neugut et al., a total of 7% of patients who presented with abdominal pain (n=113) either had carcinoma or a polyp >1 cm in size on colonoscopy [110]. It is worth mentioning that detection of the pathological process does not offer symptomatic relief in these cases. In a more recent study by Kueh and colleagues, the diagnostic yield of colonoscopy was evaluated from 2005 to 2010 in a tertiary center in New Zealand among the patients who presented with isolated abdominal pain, which accounted for 1.2% of all colonoscopies (n=2633). The diagnostic yield of colonoscopy for a cancer, adenoma, diverticulosis, or hemorrhoid in the patients with abdominal pain was significantly lower in this cohort than the yield of colonoscopy performed for other symptoms such as rectal bleeding and/or iron deficiency anemia [111].

2.5.3. *Chronic constipation*

Chronic constipation, as defined by the Rome III criteria [112], is reported to be associated with an increased risk of colon cancer in retrospective studies from the United States [113, 114], Australia [115], and Japan [116]. In contrast, no such association was found in several other studies [117-119]. Interestingly, the yield of colon cancer in colonoscopy performed for constipation alone was lower than in colonoscopy performed for routine colorectal cancer screening [120]. Patients with chronic constipation who present with alarming symptoms such as rectal bleeding, melena, iron-deficiency anemia, unintentional weight loss, or are >50 years should be evaluated with a colonoscopy to identify the etiology of the obstruction, such as cancer, stricture, or extrinsic compression. Colonoscopy can be used to treat chronic constipation based on the etiology. In patients who have undergone prior abdominal surgery, have inflammatory bowel disease, or are prone to ischemia, colonoscopy is used to dilate fibrotic strictures that lead to constipation [121-123]. Patients suffering from chronic constipation due to neurogenic bowel or acute colonic pseudo-obstruction also benefit from a percutaneous endoscopic colostomy [124]. Importantly, chronic constipation as a procedural indication for colonoscopy is independently associated with poor colon preparation requiring a rigorous amount of laxative(s) or a longer duration of preparation [125, 126].

2.5.4. *Preoperative and intraoperative localization of colonic lesions*

Colonic lesions, depending on the size and consistency, may pose some difficulty in localization by surgeons during the surgical procedure, and this could be even more difficult for laparoscopic surgeries than for open procedures. In such cases, localization of a mass or polyp of interest is very important. Preoperative colonoscopy to localize the lesion using penetrating India ink, Spot, or indocyanine green is becoming a common practice [127, 128]. The dye migrates to the peritoneal surface and allows for accurate localization. An alternative colonoscopic method of applying clips around the area of interest has also been studied, which requires intraoperative ultrasound to precisely locate the site. Both methods have their own advantages and disadvantages, such as inflammatory reaction to the dye, micro-abscesses, broad spreading of the dye in the field in smaller lesions, migration of the metallic clips, false localization, or inadvertent injection of dye in the adjacent vital structures. A recent review reported that the accuracy of endoscopic tattooing is 70-100% and the incidence of intraoperative invisible lesions is 1.6-15% [129]. The complications reviewed were mostly related to transmural injection and the spillage rates varied from 2.4 to 13% and were asymptomatic. Intraoperative colonoscopy can also be performed to localize the site of a tumor or a polypectomy site. However, intraoperative colonoscopy is an understudied field and has reported problems with insufflated air in the colon which interferes with the surgical technique.

3. Contraindications for colonoscopy (table 2)

A patient who is either unwilling to give informed consent, or has given informed consent but is uncooperative and/or unable to achieve adequate sedation for colonoscopy, should not undergo colonoscopy. Colonoscopy is also contraindicated for known or suspected colonic perforation. Medical conditions associated with a high risk of perforation such as severe toxic megacolon and fulminant colitis are considered contraindications to colonoscopy. Although not strictly contraindicated, severe IBD with deep ulceration in the rectum/distal sigmoid colon and acute diverticulitis increase the risk of colonic perforation. The risk factors for colonic perforation during colonoscopy are age > 65, low body mass index, female gender, hypoalbuminemia, inpatient status, critically ill condition, multiple morbidities, IBD, and other forms of colitis such as ischemic colitis, colonic stricture dilation, polypectomy, foreign body removal, and hemostasis such as cautery [130-132].

Patients who are or are suspected of becoming hemodynamically unstable should be medically stabilized before colonoscopy. In patients who have had a myocardial infarction, a colonoscopy performed in the first 3 weeks following the infarction can provoke an arrhythmia although the only reported complications during colonoscopy in the 30 days following an myocardial infarction are hypotension and bradycardia [133]. Adequate bowel preparation is necessary because inadequate or poor bowel preparation increases colonoscopy duration with an increase in complications as well as an increase in the number of missed adenomas and high-risk lesions [134].

Contraindications for colonoscopy:
1. Patient refusal
2. Uncooperative patients
3. Inadequate sedation
4. Known or suspected colonic perforation
5. Severe toxic megacolon and fulminant colitis
6. Clinically unstable patients
7. Recent myocardial infarction
8. Inadequate bowel preparation
9. Peritonism

Table 2. Contraindications for colonoscopy

Patients with severe abdominal pain and peritoneal signs may be at risk for possible complete obstruction or gangrenous bowel and should be evaluated by other modalities first. These patients should not undergo colonoscopy due to the risk of bowel perforation from air insufflation of a distended bowel [135]. Colonoscopic decompression of cecal volvulus, though reported, has a high failure rate. Therefore, cecal volvulus should be managed surgically [94]. Failure of endoscopic bowel detorsion, or colonic volvulus with bowel perforation, bowel infarction, or peritonitis are indications for emergent surgery [135].

Author details

Jigar Bhagatwala, Arpit Singhal, Summer Aldrugh, Muhammed Sherid, Humberto Sifuentes and Subbaramiah Sridhar*

*Address all correspondence to: jbhagatwala@gru.edu

Georgia Regents University, Augusta, GA, USA

References

[1] Wolff WI. Colonoscopy: history and development. *Am J Gastroenterol.* 1989;84(9): 1017-25. PubMed PMID: 2672788.

[2] Telford JJ. Inappropriate uses of colonoscopy. *Gastroenterol Hepatol.* 2012;8(5):342-4. PubMed PMID: 22933868; PubMed Central PMCID: PMC3424432.

[3] Committee ASoP, Pasha SF, Shergill A, Acosta RD, Chandrasekhara V, Chathadi KV, et al. The role of endoscopy in the patient with lower GI bleeding. *Gastrointest Endosc.* 2014;79(6):875-85. doi: 10.1016/j.gie.2013.10.039. PubMed PMID: 24703084.

[4] Committee ASoP, Early DS, Ben-Menachem T, Decker GA, Evans JA, Fanelli RD, et al. Appropriate use of GI endoscopy. *Gastrointest Endosc.* 2012;75(6):1127-31. doi: 10.1016/j.gie.2012.01.011. PubMed PMID: 22624807.

[5] Peytremann-Bridevaux I, Arditi C, Froehlich F, O'Malley J, Fairclough P, Le Moine O, et al. Appropriateness of colonoscopy in Europe (EPAGE II). Iron-deficiency anemia and hematochezia. *Endoscopy.* 2009;41(3):227-33. doi: 10.1055/s-0028-1119644. PubMed PMID: 19280534.

[6] Talley NJ, Jones M. Self-reported rectal bleeding in a United States community: prevalence, risk factors, and health care seeking. *Am J Gastroenterol.* 1998;93(11):2179-83. doi: 10.1111/j.1572-0241.1998.00530.x. PubMed PMID: 9820393.

[7] Caos A, Benner KG, Manier J, McCarthy DM, Blessing LD, Katon RM, et al. Colonoscopy after Golytely preparation in acute rectal bleeding. *J Clin Gastroenterol.* 1986;8(1):46-9. PubMed PMID: 3486210.

[8] Tedesco FJ, Waye JD, Raskin JB, Morris SJ, Greenwald RA. Colonoscopic evaluation of rectal bleeding: a study of 304 patients. *Ann Intern Med.* 1978;89(6):907-9. PubMed PMID: 309745.

[9] Irvine EJ, O'Connor J, Frost RA, Shorvon P, Somers S, Stevenson GW, et al. Prospective comparison of double contrast barium enema plus flexible sigmoidoscopy v colonoscopy in rectal bleeding: barium enema v colonoscopy in rectal bleeding. *Gut.* 1988;29(9):1188-93. PubMed PMID: 3273756; PubMed Central PMCID: PMC1434375.

[10] Jensen DM, Machicado GA, Jutabha R, Kovacs TO. Urgent colonoscopy for the diagnosis and treatment of severe diverticular hemorrhage. *N Eng J Med.* 2000;342(2): 78-82. doi: 10.1056/NEJM200001133420202. PubMed PMID: 10631275.

[11] Bloomfeld RS, Rockey DC, Shetzline MA. Endoscopic therapy of acute diverticular hemorrhage. *Am J Gastroenterol.* 2001;96(8):2367-72. doi: 10.1111/j.1572-0241.2001.04048.x. PubMed PMID: 11513176.

[12] Angtuaco TL, Reddy SK, Drapkin S, Harrell LE, Howden CW. The utility of urgent colonoscopy in the evaluation of acute lower gastrointestinal tract bleeding: a 2-year experience from a single center. *Am J Gastroenterol.* 2001;96(6):1782-5. doi: 10.1111/j.1572-0241.2001.03871.x. PubMed PMID: 11419829.

[13] Whitlow CB. Endoscopic treatment for lower gastrointestinal bleeding. Clinic Colon Rect Surg. 2010;23(1):31-6. doi: 10.1055/s-0030-1247855. PubMed PMID: 21286288; PubMed Central PMCID: PMC2850164.

[14] Hwang JH, Fisher DA, Ben-Menachem T, Chandrasekhara V, Chathadi K, Decker GA, et al. The role of endoscopy in the management of acute non-variceal upper GI bleeding. *Gastrointest Endosc.* 2012;75(6):1132-8. doi: 10.1016/j.gie.2012.02.033. PubMed PMID: 22624808.

[15] Espey DK, Wu XC, Swan J, Wiggins C, Jim MA, Ward E, et al. Annual report to the nation on the status of cancer, 1975-2004, featuring cancer in American Indians and Alaska Natives. *Cancer.* 2007;110(10):2119-52. doi: 10.1002/cncr.23044. PubMed PMID: 17939129.

[16] Rex DK, Johnson DA, Anderson JC, Schoenfeld PS, Burke CA, Inadomi JM, et al. American College of Gastroenterology guidelines for colorectal cancer screening 2009 [corrected]. *Am J Gastroenterol.* 2009;104(3):739-50. doi: 10.1038/ajg.2009.104. PubMed PMID: 19240699.

[17] Sung JJ, Ng SC, Chan FK, Chiu HM, Kim HS, Matsuda T, et al. An updated Asia Pacific Consensus Recommendations on colorectal cancer screening. *Gut.* 2015;64(1): 121-32. doi: 10.1136/gutjnl-2013-306503. PubMed PMID: 24647008.

[18] Frazier AL, Colditz GA, Fuchs CS, Kuntz KM. Cost-effectiveness of screening for colorectal cancer in the general population. *Jama.* 2000;284(15):1954-61. PubMed PMID: 11035892.

[19] Vijan S, Hwang EW, Hofer TP, Hayward RA. Which colon cancer screening test? A comparison of costs, effectiveness, and compliance. *Am J Med.* 2001;111(8):593-601. PubMed PMID: 11755501.

[20] Thiis-Evensen E, Hoff GS, Sauar J, Majak BM, Vatn MH. Flexible sigmoidoscopy or colonoscopy as a screening modality for colorectal adenomas in older age groups? Findings in a cohort of the normal population aged 63-72 years. *Gut.* 1999;45(6):834-9. PubMed PMID: 10562581; PubMed Central PMCID: PMC1727750.

[21] Hewitson P, Glasziou P, Irwig L, Towler B, Watson E. Screening for colorectal cancer using the faecal occult blood test, Hemoccult. *The Cochrane Database of Systematic Reviews.* 2007(1):CD001216. doi: 10.1002/14651858.CD001216.pub2. PubMed PMID: 17253456.

[22] Foutch PG, Mai H, Pardy K, DiSario JA, Manne RK, Kerr D. Flexible sigmoidoscopy may be ineffective for secondary prevention of colorectal cancer in asymptomatic, average-risk men. *Dig Dis Sci.* 1991;36(7):924-8. PubMed PMID: 2070706.

[23] Lieberman DA, Smith FW. Screening for colon malignancy with colonoscopy. *Am J Gastroenterol.* 1991;86(8):946-51. PubMed PMID: 1858758.

[24] Johns LE, Kee F, Collins BJ, Patterson CC, Houlston RS. Colorectal cancer mortality in first-degree relatives of early-onset colorectal cancer cases. *Dis Colon Rectum.* 2002;45(5):681-6. PubMed PMID: 12004220.

[25] Johns LE, Houlston RS. A systematic review and meta-analysis of familial colorectal cancer risk. *Am J Gastroenterol.* 2001;96(10):2992-3003. doi: 10.1111/j.1572-0241.2001.04677.x. PubMed PMID: 11693338.

[26] Butterworth AS, Higgins JP, Pharoah P. Relative and absolute risk of colorectal cancer for individuals with a family history: a meta-analysis. *Eur J Can.* 2006;42(2):216-27. doi: 10.1016/j.ejca.2005.09.023. PubMed PMID: 16338133.

[27] McLeod RS, Canadian Task Force on Preventive Health C. Screening strategies for colorectal cancer: a systematic review of the evidence. *Canadian J Gastroenterol = J Canadien Gastroenterol.* 2001;15(10):647-60. PubMed PMID: 11694901.

[28] Rex DK, Johnson DA, Lieberman DA, Burt RW, Sonnenberg A. Colorectal cancer prevention 2000: screening recommendations of the American College of Gastroenterology. American College of Gastroenterology. *Am J Gastroenterol.* 2000;95(4):868-77. doi: 10.1111/j.1572-0241.2000.02059.x. PubMed PMID: 10763931.

[29] Smith RA, Cokkinides V, Eyre HJ. American Cancer Society guidelines for the early detection of cancer, 2006. *CA: A Cancer Journal for Clinicians.* 2006;56(1):11-25; quiz 49-50. PubMed PMID: 16449183.

[30] Force USPST. Screening for colorectal cancer: recommendation and rationale. *Am Fam Physician*. 2002;66(12):2287-90. PubMed PMID: 12507168.

[31] Lynch HT, Smyrk T, Lynch J, Fitzgibbons R, Jr., Lanspa S, McGinn T. Update on the differential diagnosis, surveillance and management of hereditary non-polyposis colorectal cancer. *Eur J Can*. 1995;31A(7-8):1039-46. PubMed PMID: 7576988.

[32] Lieberman DA, De Garmo PL, Fleischer DE, Eisen GM, Helfand M. Patterns of endoscopy use in the United States. *Gastroenterology*. 2000;118(3):619-24. PubMed PMID: 10702214.

[33] Ladabaum U, Song K. Projected national impact of colorectal cancer screening on clinical and economic outcomes and health services demand. *Gastroenterology*. 2005;129(4):1151-62. doi: 10.1053/j.gastro.2005.07.059. PubMed PMID: 16230069.

[34] Lieberman DA, Weiss DG, Harford WV, Ahnen DJ, Provenzale D, Sontag SJ, et al. Five-year colon surveillance after screening colonoscopy. *Gastroenterology*. 2007;133(4):1077-85. doi: 10.1053/j.gastro.2007.07.006. PubMed PMID: 17698067.

[35] Leung WK, Lau JY, Suen BY, Wong GL, Chow DK, Lai LH, et al. Repeat-screening colonoscopy 5 years after normal baseline-screening colonoscopy in average-risk Chinese: a prospective study. *Am J Gastroenterol*. 2009;104(8):2028-34. doi: 10.1038/ajg.2009.202. PubMed PMID: 19455125.

[36] Brenner H, Chang-Claude J, Seiler CM, Hoffmeister M. Long-term risk of colorectal cancer after negative colonoscopy. *J Clin Oncol*: Official journal of the American Society of Clinical Oncology. 2011;29(28):3761-7. doi: 10.1200/JCO.2011.35.9307. PubMed PMID: 21876077.

[37] Brenner H, Haug U, Arndt V, Stegmaier C, Altenhofen L, Hoffmeister M. Low risk of colorectal cancer and advanced adenomas more than 10 years after negative colonoscopy. *Gastroenterology*. 2010;138(3):870-6. doi: 10.1053/j.gastro.2009.10.054. PubMed PMID: 19909750.

[38] Miller HL, Mukherjee R, Tian J, Nagar AB. Colonoscopy surveillance after polypectomy may be extended beyond five years. *J Clin Gastroenterol*. 2010;44(8):e162-6. doi: 10.1097/MCG.0b013e3181e5cd22. PubMed PMID: 20628313.

[39] Chung SJ, Kim YS, Yang SY, Song JH, Kim D, Park MJ, et al. Five-year risk for advanced colorectal neoplasia after initial colonoscopy according to the baseline risk stratification: a prospective study in 2452 asymptomatic Koreans. *Gut*. 2011;60(11):1537-43. doi: 10.1136/gut.2010.232876. PubMed PMID: 21427200.

[40] Brenner H, Chang-Claude J, Seiler CM, Rickert A, Hoffmeister M. Protection from colorectal cancer after colonoscopy: a population-based, case-control study. *Ann Internal Med*. 2011;154(1):22-30. doi: 10.7326/0003-4819-154-1-201101040-00004. PubMed PMID: 21200035.

[41] Rex DK, Kahi CJ, Levin B, Smith RA, Bond JH, Brooks D, et al. Guidelines for colonoscopy surveillance after cancer resection: a consensus update by the American Can-

cer Society and US Multi-Society Task Force on Colorectal Cancer. *CA: A Cancer Journal for Clinicians*. 2006;56(3):160-7; quiz 85-6. PubMed PMID: 16737948.

[42] Meyerhardt JA, Mangu PB, Flynn PJ, Korde L, Loprinzi CL, Minsky BD, et al. Follow-up care, surveillance protocol, and secondary prevention measures for survivors of colorectal cancer: American Society of Clinical Oncology clinical practice guideline endorsement. *J Clin Oncol*: Official journal of the American Society of Clinical Oncology. 2013;31(35):4465-70. doi: 10.1200/JCO.2013.50.7442. PubMed PMID: 24220554.

[43] Labianca R, Nordlinger B, Beretta GD, Brouquet A, Cervantes A, Group EGW. Primary colon cancer: ESMO Clinical Practice Guidelines for diagnosis, adjuvant treatment and follow-up. *Ann Oncology*: Official journal of the European Society for Medical Oncology/ESMO. 2010;21 Suppl 5:v70-7. doi: 10.1093/annonc/mdq168. PubMed PMID: 20555107.

[44] Glimelius B, Pahlman L, Cervantes A, Group EGW. Rectal cancer: ESMO Clinical Practice Guidelines for diagnosis, treatment and follow-up. *Ann Oncol*: Official journal of the European Society for Medical Oncology/ESMO. 2010;21 Suppl 5:v82-6. doi: 10.1093/annonc/mdq170. PubMed PMID: 20555109.

[45] Dignass A, Eliakim R, Magro F, Maaser C, Chowers Y, Geboes K, et al. Second European evidence-based consensus on the diagnosis and management of ulcerative colitis part 1: definitions and diagnosis. *J Crohn's Colitis*. 2012;6(10):965-90. doi: 10.1016/j.crohns.2012.09.003. PubMed PMID: 23040452.

[46] Van Assche G, Dignass A, Reinisch W, van der Woude CJ, Sturm A, De Vos M, et al. The second European evidence-based Consensus on the diagnosis and management of Crohn's disease: special situations. *J Crohn's Colitis*. 2010;4(1):63-101. doi: 10.1016/j.crohns.2009.09.009. PubMed PMID: 21122490.

[47] Mowat C, Cole A, Windsor A, Ahmad T, Arnott I, Driscoll R, et al. Guidelines for the management of inflammatory bowel disease in adults. *Gut*. 2011;60(5):571-607. doi: 10.1136/gut.2010.224154. PubMed PMID: 21464096.

[48] Leighton JA, Shen B, Baron TH, Adler DG, Davila R, Egan JV, et al. ASGE guideline: endoscopy in the diagnosis and treatment of inflammatory bowel disease. *Gastrointest Endosc*. 2006;63(4):558-65. doi: 10.1016/j.gie.2006.02.005. PubMed PMID: 16564852.

[49] Horsthuis K, Stokkers PC, Stoker J. Detection of inflammatory bowel disease: diagnostic performance of cross-sectional imaging modalities. *Abdom Imaging*. 2008;33(4): 407-16. doi: 10.1007/s00261-007-9276-3. PubMed PMID: 17619923; PubMed Central PMCID: PMC2386533.

[50] Marshall JK, Cawdron R, Zealley I, Riddell RH, Somers S, Irvine EJ. Prospective comparison of small bowel meal with pneumocolon versus ileo-colonoscopy for the diagnosis of ileal Crohn's disease. *Am J Gastroenterol*. 2004;99(7):1321-9. doi: 10.1111/j.1572-0241.2004.30499.x. PubMed PMID: 15233672.

[51] Richards ME, Rickert RR, Nance FC. Crohn's disease-associated carcinoma. A poorly recognized complication of inflammatory bowel disease. *Ann Surg*. 1989;209(6): 764-73. PubMed PMID: 2543338; PubMed Central PMCID: PMC1494126.

[52] Ekbom A, Helmick C, Zack M, Adami HO. Increased risk of large-bowel cancer in Crohn's disease with colonic involvement. *Lancet*. 1990;336(8711):357-9. PubMed PMID: 1975343.

[53] Farraye FA, Odze RD, Eaden J, Itzkowitz SH. AGA technical review on the diagnosis and management of colorectal neoplasia in inflammatory bowel disease. *Gastroenterology*. 2010;138(2):746-74, 74 e1-4; quiz e12-3. doi: 10.1053/j.gastro.2009.12.035. PubMed PMID: 20141809.

[54] Friedman S, Rubin PH, Bodian C, Goldstein E, Harpaz N, Present DH. Screening and surveillance colonoscopy in chronic Crohn's colitis. *Gastroenterology*. 2001;120(4): 820-6. PubMed PMID: 11231935.

[55] Maykel JA, Hagerman G, Mellgren AF, Li SY, Alavi K, Baxter NN, et al. Crohn's colitis: the incidence of dysplasia and adenocarcinoma in surgical patients. *Dis Colon Rectum*. 2006;49(7):950-7. doi: 10.1007/s10350-006-0555-9. PubMed PMID: 16729218.

[56] Jess T, Loftus EV, Jr., Velayos FS, Harmsen WS, Zinsmeister AR, Smyrk TC, et al. Risk of intestinal cancer in inflammatory bowel disease: a population-based study from olmsted county, Minnesota. *Gastroenterology*. 2006;130(4):1039-46. doi: 10.1053/j.gastro.2005.12.037. PubMed PMID: 16618397.

[57] Karlen P, Kornfeld D, Brostrom O, Lofberg R, Persson PG, Ekbom A. Is colonoscopic surveillance reducing colorectal cancer mortality in ulcerative colitis? A population based case control study. *Gut*. 1998;42(5):711-4. PubMed PMID: 9659169; PubMed Central PMCID: PMC1727094.

[58] Lutgens MW, Oldenburg B, Siersema PD, van Bodegraven AA, Dijkstra G, Hommes DW, et al. Colonoscopic surveillance improves survival after colorectal cancer diagnosis in inflammatory bowel disease. *Brit J Can*. 2009;101(10):1671-5. doi: 10.1038/sj.bjc.6605359. PubMed PMID: 19826420; PubMed Central PMCID: PMC2778537.

[59] Ananthakrishnan AN, Cagan A, Cai T, Gainer VS, Shaw SY, Churchill S, et al. Colonoscopy is associated with a reduced risk for colon cancer and mortality in patients with inflammatory bowel diseases. *Clin Gastroenterol Hepatol*: Official clinical practice journal of the American Gastroenterological Association. 2014. doi: 10.1016/j.cgh.2014.07.018. PubMed PMID: 25041865; PubMed Central PMCID: PMC4297589.

[60] Cairns SR, Scholefield JH, Steele RJ, Dunlop MG, Thomas HJ, Evans GD, et al. Guidelines for colorectal cancer screening and surveillance in moderate and high risk groups (update from 2002). *Gut*. 2010;59(5):666-89. doi: 10.1136/gut.2009.179804. PubMed PMID: 20427401.

[61] Van Assche G, Dignass A, Bokemeyer B, Danese S, Gionchetti P, Moser G, et al. Second European evidence-based consensus on the diagnosis and management of ulcer-

ative colitis part 3: special situations. *J Crohn's Colitis*. 2013;7(1):1-33. doi: 10.1016/j.crohns.2012.09.005. PubMed PMID: 23040453.

[62] Cancer Council Australia Colonoscopy Surveillance Working Party. Clinical practice guidelines for surveillance colonoscopy – in adenoma follow-up; following curative resection of colorectal cancer; and for cancer surveillance in inflammatory bowel disease. Sydney (Australia): Cancer Council Australia; 2011 Dec. 144 p. Available from: http://www.guideline.gov/content.aspx?id=47635.

[63] Lasson A, Kilander A, Stotzer PO. Diagnostic yield of colonoscopy based on symptoms. *Scand J Gastroenterol*. 2008;43(3):356-62. PubMed PMID: 18938663.

[64] Shah RJ, Fenoglio-Preiser C, Bleau BL, Giannella RA. Usefulness of colonoscopy with biopsy in the evaluation of patients with chronic diarrhea. *Am J Gastroenterol*. 2001;96(4):1091-5. doi: 10.1111/j.1572-0241.2001.03745.x. PubMed PMID: 11316152.

[65] Tanaka M, Mazzoleni G, Riddell RH. Distribution of collagenous colitis: utility of flexible sigmoidoscopy. *Gut*. 1992;33(1):65-70. PubMed PMID: 1740280; PubMed Central PMCID: PMC1373867.

[66] McHugh JB, Appelman HD, McKenna BJ. The diagnostic value of endoscopic terminal ileum biopsies. *Am J Gastroenterol*. 2007;102(5):1084-9. doi: 10.1111/j.1572-0241.2007.01194.x. PubMed PMID: 17391315.

[67] Kearney DJ, Steuerwald M, Koch J, Cello JP. A prospective study of endoscopy in HIV-associated diarrhea. *Am J Gastroenterol*. 1999;94(3):596-602. doi: 10.1111/j.1572-0241.1999.00920.x. PubMed PMID: 10086637.

[68] Khan K, Schwarzenberg SJ, Sharp H, Jessurun J, Gulbahce HE, Defor T, et al. Diagnostic endoscopy in children after hematopoietic stem cell transplantation. *Gastrointest Endosc*. 2006;64(3):379-85; quiz 89-92. doi: 10.1016/j.gie.2005.08.040. PubMed PMID: 16923486.

[69] Saito Y, Fukuzawa M, Matsuda T, Fukunaga S, Sakamoto T, Uraoka T, et al. Clinical outcome of endoscopic submucosal dissection versus endoscopic mucosal resection of large colorectal tumors as determined by curative resection. *Surg Endosc*. 2010;24(2):343-52. doi: 10.1007/s00464-009-0562-8. PubMed PMID: 19517168.

[70] Tajika M, Niwa Y, Bhatia V, Kondo S, Tanaka T, Mizuno N, et al. Comparison of endoscopic submucosal dissection and endoscopic mucosal resection for large colorectal tumors. *Eur J Gastroenterol Hepatol*. 2011;23(11):1042-9. doi: 10.1097/MEG.0b013e32834aa47b. PubMed PMID: 21869682.

[71] Isomoto H, Nishiyama H, Yamaguchi N, Fukuda E, Ishii H, Ikeda K, et al. Clinicopathological factors associated with clinical outcomes of endoscopic submucosal dissection for colorectal epithelial neoplasms. *Endoscopy*. 2009;41(8):679-83. doi: 10.1055/s-0029-1214979. PubMed PMID: 19670135.

[72] Yoshida N, Naito Y, Sakai K, Sumida Y, Kanemasa K, Inoue K, et al. Outcome of endoscopic submucosal dissection for colorectal tumors in elderly people. *Int J Colorectal Dis*. 2010;25(4):455-61. doi: 10.1007/s00384-009-0841-9. PubMed PMID: 19921221.

[73] Yoshida N, Wakabayashi N, Kanemasa K, Sumida Y, Hasegawa D, Inoue K, et al. Endoscopic submucosal dissection for colorectal tumors: technical difficulties and rate of perforation. *Endoscopy*. 2009;41(9):758-61. doi: 10.1055/s-0029-1215028. PubMed PMID: 19746316.

[74] oshida N, Yagi N, Naito Y, Yoshikawa T. Safe procedure in endoscopic submucosal dissection for colorectal tumors focused on preventing complications. *World J Gastroenterol: WJG*. 2010;16(14):1688-95. PubMed PMID: 20379999; PubMed Central PMCID: PMC2852815.

[75] Savides TJ, Jensen DM. Colonoscopic hemostasis for recurrent diverticular hemorrhage associated with a visible vessel: a report of three cases. *Gastrointest Endosc*. 1994;40(1):70-3. PubMed PMID: 8163141.

[76] Binmoeller KF, Thonke F, Soehendra N. Endoscopic hemoclip treatment for gastrointestinal bleeding. *Endoscopy*. 1993;25(2):167-70. doi: 10.1055/s-2007-1010277. PubMed PMID: 8491134.

[77] Santos JC, Jr., Aprilli F, Guimaraes AS, Rocha JJ. Angiodysplasia of the colon: endoscopic diagnosis and treatment. *Brit J Surg*. 1988;75(3):256-8. PubMed PMID: 3258173.

[78] Sagar J. Colorectal stents for the management of malignant colonic obstructions. *The Cochrane Database of Systematic Reviews*. 2011(11):CD007378. doi: 10.1002/14651858.CD007378.pub2. PubMed PMID: 22071835.

[79] Frago R, Ramirez E, Millan M, Kreisler E, del Valle E, Biondo S. Current management of acute malignant large bowel obstruction: a systematic review. *Am J Surg*. 2014;207(1):127-38. doi: 10.1016/j.amjsurg.2013.07.027. PubMed PMID: 24124659.

[80] Cheung DY, Kim JY, Hong SP, Jung MK, Ye BD, Kim SG, et al. Outcome and safety of self-expandable metallic stents for malignant colon obstruction: a Korean multicenter randomized prospective study. *Surg Endosc*. 2012;26(11):3106-13. doi: 10.1007/s00464-012-2300-x. PubMed PMID: 22609981.

[81] Varadarajulu S, Roy A, Lopes T, Drelichman ER, Kim M. Endoscopic stenting versus surgical colostomy for the management of malignant colonic obstruction: comparison of hospital costs and clinical outcomes. *Surg Endosc*. 2011;25(7):2203-9. doi: 10.1007/s00464-010-1523-y. PubMed PMID: 21293882; PubMed Central PMCID: PMC3116133.

[82] Kavanagh DO, Nolan B, Judge C, Hyland JM, Mulcahy HE, O'Connell PR, et al. A comparative study of short- and medium-term outcomes comparing emergent surgery and stenting as a bridge to surgery in patients with acute malignant colonic ob-

struction. *Dis Colon Rectum*. 2013;56(4):433-40. doi: 10.1097/DCR.0b013e3182760506. PubMed PMID: 23478610.

[83] van Hooft JE, Bemelman WA, Oldenburg B, Marinelli AW, Lutke Holzik MF, Grubben MJ, et al. Colonic stenting versus emergency surgery for acute left-sided malignant colonic obstruction: a multicentre randomised trial. *Lancet Oncol*. 2011;12(4): 344-52. doi: 10.1016/S1470-2045(11)70035-3. PubMed PMID: 21398178.

[84] Gevers AM, Macken E, Hiele M, Rutgeerts P. Endoscopic laser therapy for palliation of patients with distal colorectal carcinoma: analysis of factors influencing long-term outcome. *Gastrointest Endosc*. 2000;51(5):580-5. PubMed PMID: 10805846.

[85] Solecki R, Zajac A, Richter P, Szura M. Bifocal esophageal and rectal cancer palliatively treated with argon plasma coagulation. *Surgical Endosc*. 2004;18(2):346. doi: 10.1007/s00464-003-4232-y. PubMed PMID: 15106621.

[86] Baumhoer D, Armbrust T, Ramadori G. Nonsurgical treatment of the primary tumor in four consecutive cases of metastasized colorectal carcinoma. *Endoscopy*. 2005;37(12):1232-6. doi: 10.1055/s-2005-870225. PubMed PMID: 16329023.

[87] Saunders MD. Acute colonic pseudo-obstruction. *Best Pract Res Clin Gastroenterol*. 2007;21(4):671-87. doi: 10.1016/j.bpg.2007.03.001. PubMed PMID: 17643908.

[88] Tsirline VB, Zemlyak AY, Avery MJ, Colavita PD, Christmas AB, Heniford BT, et al. Colonoscopy is superior to neostigmine in the treatment of Ogilvie's syndrome. *Am J Surg*. 2012;204(6):849-55; discussion 55. doi: 10.1016/j.amjsurg.2012.05.006. PubMed PMID: 23021196.

[89] Renzulli P, Maurer CA, Netzer P, Buchler MW. Preoperative colonoscopic derotation is beneficial in acute colonic volvulus. *Dig Surg*. 2002;19(3):223-9. PubMed PMID: 12119526.

[90] Swenson BR, Kwaan MR, Burkart NE, Wang Y, Madoff RD, Rothenberger DA, et al. Colonic volvulus: presentation and management in metropolitan Minnesota, United States. *Dis Colon Rectum*. 2012;55(4):444-9. doi: 10.1097/DCR.0b013e3182404b3d. PubMed PMID: 22426269.

[91] Halabi WJ, Jafari MD, Kang CY, Nguyen VQ, Carmichael JC, Mills S, et al. Colonic volvulus in the United States: trends, outcomes, and predictors of mortality. *Ann Surg*. 2014;259(2):293-301. doi: 10.1097/SLA.0b013e31828c88ac. PubMed PMID: 23511842.

[92] Oren D, Atamanalp SS, Aydinli B, Yildirgan MI, Basoglu M, Polat KY, et al. An algorithm for the management of sigmoid colon volvulus and the safety of primary resection: experience with 827 cases. *Dis Colon Rectum*. 2007;50(4):489-97. doi: 10.1007/s10350-006-0821-x. PubMed PMID: 17205203.

[93] Ballantyne GH. Review of sigmoid volvulus: history and results of treatment. *Dis Colon Rectum*. 1982;25(5):494-501. PubMed PMID: 7047106.

[94] Madiba TE, Thomson SR. The management of cecal volvulus. *Dis Colon Rectum.* 2002;45(2):264-7. PubMed PMID: 11852342.

[95] Hassan C, Zullo A, De Francesco V, Ierardi E, Giustini M, Pitidis A, et al. Systematic review: Endoscopic dilatation in Crohn's disease. *Alim Pharmacol Therapeut.* 2007;26(11-12):1457-64. doi: 10.1111/j.1365-2036.2007.03532.x. PubMed PMID: 17903236.

[96] Ramboer C, Verhamme M, Dhondt E, Huys S, Van Eygen K, Vermeire L. Endoscopic treatment of stenosis in recurrent Crohn's disease with balloon dilation combined with local corticosteroid injection. *Gastrointest Endosc.* 1995;42(3):252-5. PubMed PMID: 7498692.

[97] Lucha PA, Jr., Fticsar JE, Francis MJ. The strictured anastomosis: successful treatment by corticosteroid injections – report of three cases and review of the literature. *Dis Colon Rectum.* 2005;48(4):862-5. doi: 10.1007/s10350-004-0838-y. PubMed PMID: 15747075.

[98] East JE, Brooker JC, Rutter MD, Saunders BP. A pilot study of intrastricture steroid versus placebo injection after balloon dilatation of Crohn's strictures. *Clin Gastroenterol Hepatol*: The official clinical practice journal of the American Gastroenterological Association. 2007;5(9):1065-9. doi: 10.1016/j.cgh.2007.04.013. PubMed PMID: 17627903.

[99] Brooker JC, Beckett CG, Saunders BP, Benson MJ. Long-acting steroid injection after endoscopic dilation of anastomotic Crohn's strictures may improve the outcome: a retrospective case series. *Endoscopy.* 2003;35(4):333-7. doi: 10.1055/s-2003-38145. PubMed PMID: 12664391.

[100] Brandimarte G, Tursi A, Gasbarrini G. Endoscopic treatment of benign anastomotic colorectal stenosis with electrocautery. *Endoscopy.* 2000;32(6):461-3. doi: 10.1055/s-2000-651. PubMed PMID: 10863912.

[101] Hagiwara A, Togawa T, Yamasaki J, Shirasu M, Sakakura C, Yamagishi H. Endoscopic incision and balloon dilatation for cicatricial anastomotic strictures. *Hepatogastroenterology.* 1999;46(26):997-9. PubMed PMID: 10370654.

[102] Koornstra JJ, Weersma RK. Management of rectal foreign bodies: description of a new technique and clinical practice guidelines. World journal of gastroenterology : WJG. 2008;14(27):4403-6. PubMed PMID: 18666334; PubMed Central PMCID: PMC2731197.

[103] Goldberg JE, Steele SR. Rectal foreign bodies. *Surg Clin N Am.* 2010;90(1):173-84, Table of Contents. doi: 10.1016/j.suc.2009.10.004. PubMed PMID: 20109641.

[104] Singaporewalla RM, Tan DE, Tan TK. Use of endoscopic snare to extract a large rectosigmoid foreign body with review of literature. *Surgical Laparosc, Endosc Percut Tech.* 2007;17(2):145-8. doi: 10.1097/SLE.0b013e318045bf1a. PubMed PMID: 17450100.

[105] Humes D, Lobo DN. Removal of a rectal foreign body by using a Foley catheter passed through a rigid sigmoidoscope. *Gastrointestinal Endosc.* 2005;62(4):610. PubMed PMID: 16185979.

[106] Billi P, Bassi M, Ferrara F, Biscardi A, Villani S, Baldoni F, et al. Endoscopic removal of a large rectal foreign body using a large balloon dilator: report of a case and description of the technique. *Endoscopy.* 2010;42 Suppl 2:E238. doi: 10.1055/s-0030-1255573. PubMed PMID: 20931459.

[107] Rex DK, Lieberman D, Acg. ACG colorectal cancer prevention action plan: update on CT-colonography. *Am Journal of Gastroenterol.* 2006;101(7):1410-3. doi: 10.1111/j.1572-0241.2006.00585.x. PubMed PMID: 16863539.

[108] Rockey DC, Barish M, Brill JV, Cash BD, Fletcher JG, Sharma P, et al. Standards for gastroenterologists for performing and interpreting diagnostic computed tomographic colonography. *Gastroenterology.* 2007;133(3):1005-24. doi: 10.1053/j.gastro.2007.06.001. PubMed PMID: 17678924.

[109] Zalis ME, Barish MA, Choi JR, Dachman AH, Fenlon HM, Ferrucci JT, et al. CT colonography reporting and data system: a consensus proposal. *Radiology.* 2005;236(1):3-9. doi: 10.1148/radiol.2361041926. PubMed PMID: 15987959.

[110] Neugut AI, Garbowski GC, Waye JD, Forde KA, Treat MR, Tsai JL, et al. Diagnostic yield of colorectal neoplasia with colonoscopy for abdominal pain, change in bowel habits, and rectal bleeding. *Am J Gastroenterol.* 1993;88(8):1179-83. PubMed PMID: 8338084.

[111] Kueh SH, Zhou L, Walmsley RS. The diagnostic yield of colonoscopy in patients with isolated abdominal pain. *N Zea Med J.* 2013;126(1382):36-44. PubMed PMID: 24154768.

[112] Longstreth GF, Thompson WG, Chey WD, Houghton LA, Mearin F, Spiller RC. Functional bowel disorders. *Gastroenterology.* 2006;130(5):1480-91. doi: 10.1053/j.gastro.2005.11.061. PubMed PMID: 16678561.

[113] Roberts MC, Millikan RC, Galanko JA, Martin C, Sandler RS. Constipation, laxative use, and colon cancer in a North Carolina population. *Am J Gastroenterol.* 2003;98(4):857-64. doi: 10.1111/j.1572-0241.2003.07386.x. PubMed PMID: 12738468.

[114] Jacobs EJ, White E. Constipation, laxative use, and colon cancer among middle-aged adults. *Epidemiology.* 1998;9(4):385-91. PubMed PMID: 9647901.

[115] Kune GA, Kune S, Field B, Watson LF. The role of chronic constipation, diarrhea, and laxative use in the etiology of large-bowel cancer. Data from the Melbourne colorectal cancer study. *Dis Colon Rectum.* 1988;31(7):507-12. PubMed PMID: 3391059.

[116] Watanabe T, Nakaya N, Kurashima K, Kuriyama S, Tsubono Y, Tsuji I. Constipation, laxative use and risk of colorectal cancer: The Miyagi Cohort Study. *Eur J Can.* 2004;40(14):2109-15. doi: 10.1016/j.ejca.2004.06.014. PubMed PMID: 15341986.

[117] Dukas L, Willett WC, Colditz GA, Fuchs CS, Rosner B, Giovannucci EL. Prospective study of bowel movement, laxative use, and risk of colorectal cancer among women. *Am J Epidemiol.* 2000;151(10):958-64. PubMed PMID: 10853634.

[118] Anderson JC, Lacy BE. Editorial: Constipation and colorectal cancer risk: a continuing conundrum. *Am J Gastroenterol.* 2014;109(10):1650-2. doi: 10.1038/ajg.2014.292. PubMed PMID: 25287089.

[119] Power AM, Talley NJ, Ford AC. Association between constipation and colorectal cancer: systematic review and meta-analysis of observational studies. *Am J Gastroenterol.* 2013;108(6):894-903; quiz 4. doi: 10.1038/ajg.2013.52. PubMed PMID: 23481143.

[120] Obusez EC, Lian L, Kariv R, Burke CA, Shen B. Diagnostic yield of colonoscopy for constipation as the sole indication. *Colorect Dis*: The official journal of the Association of Coloproctology of Great Britain and Ireland. 2012;14(5):585-91. doi: 10.1111/j.1463-1318.2011.02664.x. PubMed PMID: 21689337.

[121] Virgilio C, Cosentino S, Favara C, Russo V, Russo A. Endoscopic treatment of postoperative colonic strictures using an achalasia dilator: short-term and long-term results. *Endoscopy.* 1995;27(3):219-22. doi: 10.1055/s-2007-1005674. PubMed PMID: 7664698.

[122] Sabate JM, Villarejo J, Bouhnik Y, Allez M, Gornet JM, Vahedi K, et al. Hydrostatic balloon dilatation of Crohn's strictures. *Alim Pharmacol Therapeut.* 2003;18(4):409-13. PubMed PMID: 12940926.

[123] Morini S, Hassan C, Lorenzetti R, Zullo A, Cerro P, Winn S, et al. Long-term outcome of endoscopic pneumatic dilatation in Crohn's disease. *Dig Liver Dis*: Official journal of the Italian Society of Gastroenterology and the Italian Association for the Study of the Liver. 2003;35(12):893-7. PubMed PMID: 14703886.

[124] Ramage JI, Jr., Baron TH. Percutaneous endoscopic cecostomy: a case series. *Gastrointest Endosc.* 2003;57(6):752-5. doi: 10.1067/mge.2003.197. PubMed PMID: 12709715.

[125] Ness RM, Manam R, Hoen H, Chalasani N. Predictors of inadequate bowel preparation for colonoscopy. Am J Gastroenterol. 2001;96(6):1797-802. doi: 10.1111/j.1572-0241.2001.03874.x. PubMed PMID: 11419832.

[126] Van Dongen M. Enhancing bowel preparation for colonoscopy: an integrative review. *Gastroenterol Nurs*: The official journal of the Society of Gastroenterology Nurses and Associates. 2012;35(1):36-44. doi: 10.1097/SGA.0b013e3182403413. PubMed PMID: 22306728.

[127] Committee AT, Kethu SR, Banerjee S, Desilets D, Diehl DL, Farraye FA, et al. Endoscopic tattooing. *Gastrointest Endosc.* 2010;72(4):681-5. doi: 10.1016/j.gie.2010.06.020. PubMed PMID: 20883844.

[128] Park JW, Sohn DK, Hong CW, Han KS, Choi DH, Chang HJ, et al. The usefulness of preoperative colonoscopic tattooing using a saline test injection method with pre-

packaged sterile India ink for localization in laparoscopic colorectal surgery. *Surg Endosc.* 2008;22(2):501-5. doi: 10.1007/s00464-007-9495-2. PubMed PMID: 17704874.

[129] Trakarnsanga A, Akaraviputh T. Endoscopic tattooing of colorectal lesions: Is it a risk-free procedure? *World J Gastrointest Endosc.* 2011;3(12):256-60. doi: 10.4253/wjge.v3.i12.256. PubMed PMID: 22195235; PubMed Central PMCID: PMC3244942.

[130] Hamdani U, Naeem R, Haider F, Bansal P, Komar M, Diehl DL, et al. Risk factors for colonoscopic perforation: a population-based study of 80118 cases. *World J Gastroenterol: WJG.* 2013;19(23):3596-601. doi: 10.3748/wjg.v19.i23.3596. PubMed PMID: 23801860; PubMed Central PMCID: PMC3691036.

[131] Polter DE. Risk of colon perforation during colonoscopy at Baylor University Medical Center. *Proceedings.* 2015;28(1):3-6. PubMed PMID: 25552784; PubMed Central PMCID: PMC4264696.

[132] Rex DK, Petrini JL, Baron TH, Chak A, Cohen J, Deal SE, et al. Quality indicators for colonoscopy. *Am J Gastroenterol.* 2006;101(4):873-85. doi: 10.1111/j.1572-0241.2006.00673.x. PubMed PMID: 16635231.

[133] Cappell MS. Safety and efficacy of colonoscopy after myocardial infarction: an analysis of 100 study patients and 100 control patients at two tertiary cardiac referral hospitals. *Gastrointest Endosc.* 2004;60(6):901-9. PubMed PMID: 15605004.

[134] Chokshi RV, Hovis CE, Hollander T, Early DS, Wang JS. Prevalence of missed adenomas in patients with inadequate bowel preparation on screening colonoscopy. *Gastrointest Endosc.* 2012;75(6):1197-203. doi: 10.1016/j.gie.2012.01.005. PubMed PMID: 22381531.

[135] Committee ASoP, Harrison ME, Anderson MA, Appalaneni V, Banerjee S, Ben-Menachem T, et al. The role of endoscopy in the management of patients with known and suspected colonic obstruction and pseudo-obstruction. Gastrointest Endosc. 2010;71(4):669-79. doi: 10.1016/j.gie.2009.11.027. PubMed PMID: 20363408.

Chapter 4

Epidemiology of Colorectal Cancer — Incidence, Lifetime Risk Factors Statistics and Temporal Trends

Camille Thélin and Sanjay Sikka

Additional information is available at the end of the chapter

http://dx.doi.org/10.5772/61945

Abstract

Colorectal cancer is a major cause of morbidity and mortality in the entire world. Among cancers that affect both men and women, it accounts for >8% of all cancer incidence, making it the third most common cancer worldwide (behind lung and breast cancer). There were an estimated 14.1 million cancer cases around the world in 2012-last data available; 7.4 million were in men and 6.7 million in women. Of that, nearly 1.4 million new cases were from colorectal cancer. And, it has consistently been shown that the developed world carries the majority of the burden (Australia, New Zealand, Canada, the United States and parts of Western Europe), likely due to similarity in lifestyles and diets.

Keywords: Colon cancer epidemiology, colorectal cancer, SEER

1. Introduction

Colorectal cancer is a major cause of morbidity and mortality in the entire world. It has consistently been shown that the developed world carries the majority of the burden — this includes Australia, New Zealand, Canada, the United States and parts of Western Europe — likely due to similarity in lifestyles and diets. [9, 12]

Among cancers that affect both men and women, colorectal cancer accounts for >8% of all cancer incidence, making it the third most common cancer worldwide, behind lung and breast cancer (Table 1). [1]

	Cancer	New cases diagnosed in 2012 (1,000s)	Percent of all cancers*
Worldwide			
1	Lung	1,825	13.0
2	Breast	1,677	11.9
3	**Colorectal**	**1,361**	**9.7**
Men			
1	Lung	1,242	16.7
2	Prostate	1,112	15.0
3	**Colorectal**	**746**	**10.0**
Women			
1	Breast	1,677	25.2
2	**Colorectal**	**614**	**9.2**
3	**Lung**	**583**	**8.8**

*Excludes basal cell and squamous cell skin cancers and *in situ* carcinoma except urinary bladder. Source: GLOBOCAN 2012 v1.1, "Cancer Incidence and Mortality Worldwide"

Table 1. Cancer Incidence Worldwide

There were an estimated 14.1 million cancer cases around the world in 2012. [1] Of those cancers, 7.4 million were in men, while 6.7 million were in women. [1] Nearly, 1.4 million of those new cancer cases were from colorectal cancer. [1]

In the United States, the breakdown between genders is similar. Colorectal cancer is the third most common cancer in both women and men (after breast and prostate cancer, respectively, and lung cancer). Among both gender groups, it is the second leading cause of cancer deaths (behind lung cancer), with peak incidence being in the seventh decade of life. [24] In 2015, it is estimated that there will be 848,200 new cases of cancer among men and 810,000 among women in 2015 (Table 2). [2] Of those new cancer cases, 8% will comprise of colon and rectal cancer, with an estimated 69,090 in men and 63,610 in females. [2]

Men 848,200	Male	Female	Women 810,000
Prostate	26%	29%	Breast
Lung & bronchus	14%	13%	Lung & bronchus
Colon & rectum	**8% (69,090)**	**8% (63,610)**	**Colon & rectum**
Urinary bladder	7%	7%	Uterine corpus

http://dx.doi.org/10.5772/61945

Men 848,200	Male	Female	Women 810,000
Melanoma of skin	5%	6%	Thyroid
Non-Hodgkin lymphoma	5%	4%	Non-Hodgkin lymphoma
Kidney & renal pelvis	5%	4%	Melanoma of skin
Oral cavity & pharynx	4%	4%	Pancreas
Leukemia	4%	3%	Leukemia
Liver & intrahepatic bile duct	3%	3%	Kidney & renal pelvis
All other sites	21%	21%	All other sites

*Excludes basal cell and squamous cell skin cancers and *in situ* carcinoma except urinary bladder.

Source: American Cancer Society, —Cancer Facts and Figures 2015.|| Projected cases are based on incidence data during 1995-2011 from 49 states and the District of Columbia, as reported by the North American Association of

Central Cancer Registries (NAACCR).

Note: Estimates should not be compared with those from previous years.

Table 2. Estimated New Cancer Cases* in the U.S. in 2015

2. Clinical presentation of colorectal cancer

The importance of screening is crucial as most early-stage colorectal cancer does not typically have symptoms. In fact, colorectal cancer may be quiescently growing for as long as 5 years before symptoms appear.

2.1. Signs and symptoms

Symptoms can be specific, such as abdominal discomfort and alarming changes in bowel movements (i.e., hematochezia, diarrhea, or obstruction). More often than not, however, symptoms are usually nonspecific, such as fatigue, weight loss, and/or changes in digestion. As such, even those with some type of symptoms have been misdiagnosed with other benign conditions. These benign conditions include examples such as diverticular disease, inflammatory bowel syndrome, or hemorrhoids. [4]

The major biochemical sign is that of new onset anemia. In fact, in those older than 40 years old, a new onset anemia — specifically hypochromic and microcytic — should prompt evaluation for colorectal cancer.

2.2. Right-sided colon cancers

Symptoms depend somewhat on the site of the tumor. In general, **right-sided colon cancers** are usually detected at an advanced stage with severe symptoms. In general, the right-sided colon cancers are commonly larger, producing vague abdominal discomfort and sometimes a palpable mass. [4, 5] Obstruction is rarely a presenting symptom, as the diameter of the right colon is larger than the left colon. [4] If the tumor involves the cecum, however, it could block the ileocecal valve causing small bowel obstruction.

Those with right-sided colon cancers are significantly older and are predominantly women (46% women versus 38% men). [6] Because of higher rates of comorbidities, survival is worse in those with right-sided carcinomas.

2.3. Left-sided colon cancers and rectal cancers

In comparison, **left-sided colon cancers and rectal cancers** tend to arise in younger, male populations with high-incidence risk. [7, 8] Cancers involving this portion of the bowel produce symptoms that range from obstruction to tenesmus, to alternating constipation and diarrhea with pencil-thin stools. [4] Often, there is blood witnessed either in the stool or coating the stool, in comparison to the right-sided colon cancers. Similarly, rectal cancers can cause obstruction and similar types of bowel movement changes as the left-sided carcinomas.

3. Risk factors of colorectal cancer

There are both modifiable and nonmodifiable risk factors associated with the incidence of colorectal cancer (Table 3).

Modifiable Risk Factors	Nonmodifiable Risk Factors
Diet	Age (≥50 years old)
Physical activity	Personal history of adenomatous colonic polyps
Body weight	Family history of colorectal cancer
Social behaviors (i.e., alcohol and cigarette smoking)	Hereditary polyposis conditions
	Personal history of inflammatory bowel disease (IBD)

Table 3. Factors Associated with Higher Risk of Colon and Rectal Cancer

Modifiable risk factors include diet, physical activity, weight, cigarette-smoking, and alcohol intake. [9] Other modifiable risk factors include low calcium content, low selenium content, and very low salt intake. [10] Occupational hazards, such as asbestos-exposure, have been linked to increased risk of colorectal cancer when compared to the rest of the general population. [10]

http://dx.doi.org/10.5772/61945

Socioeconomic factors, along with access to (and use of) health care services, are also important contributing risk factors. In fact, there is a disproportionately high incidence of colorectal cancers in low socioeconomic status populations. [11]

Nonmodifiable risk factors associated with higher risk of colorectal cancer include increasing age, personal history of adenomatous polyps, personal history of inflammatory bowel disease, genetic inheritance, race/ethnicity, and gender. [9] Unlike modifiable risk factors that could theoretically have been avoided, these risk factors are not considered part of the "environmental nature" of this disease. Thus, they are not controllable. They do, however, play an important role in screening and identifying susceptible patients.

3.1. Modifiable risk factors: Diet

Diets associated with high incidence of colorectal cancer include diets with high consumption of red or processed meat, diets high in fat, beer-drinking, diets low in calcium intake, and diets low in whole-grain fiber, fruits and vegetables. [9] This represents a typical "Western diet."

On average, 40–45% of Western diets have total caloric intake made up from fatty foods (including meat products), while fat only accounts for about 10–15% of dietary makeup in lower-risk populations — China, India, and parts of Africa and South America. Consequently, it has been shown that the developed world carries the majority of the burden (Australia, New Zealand, Canada, the United States and parts of Western Europe), [9, 12] likely due to similarity in lifestyles and diets.

The hypothesis behind dietary fat as a risk factor is that the fat enhances hepatic cholesterol and bile acid synthesis resulting in increased sterols in the colon. [4] Those sterols are then converted into secondary bile acids, cholesterol metabolites, and potentially toxic metabolic compounds. [4, 13]

While the exact pathogenesis remains unknown, what is known is that these sterols and bile acid metabolites cause damage to colonic mucosa, thus enhancing proliferative activity which could lead to dysplasia. [4, 13] This has been demonstrated in animal models, where animals fed polyunsaturated and saturated fats have higher numbers of adenocarcinoma than those on a low-fat diet. [4] This has also been shown in human population studies where those with colorectal cancer tend to have higher fecal bile acid levels, [4] while a recent meta-analysis has shown that consumption of red meat and processed meat is positively associated with risk of both colon — particularly the descending and sigmoid colon — and rectal cancer. [14]

The "Western diet" also comprises of lower amounts of fiber intake. Multiple epidemiology studies have shown a geographical difference of lower colorectal cancer incidence rates in places with higher fiber intake. [9] It is even postulated that due to the ability of fiber to change the colonic pH, carcinogenesis may be impeded. [4, 9]

Dietary fiber also increases fecal bulk, thus diluting the aforementioned carcinogenic compounds and reducing transit time and mucosal contact. In fact, fiber has been found to decrease the concentration of sterol and bile acid metabolites that could be implicated in creating carcinogenic compounds. [4] Again, this has been demonstrated in animal models, where increased fiber intake led to decreased concentration of specific bacterial metabolic enzymes that could be implicated in creating carcinogenic compounds. [4] Unfortunately, for all its experimentally demonstrative protective roles, increased fiber supplementation has been unable to prevent adenoma recurrence in several randomized-controlled trials.

3.2. Modifiable risk factors: Physical activity and body weight

Other modifiable risk factors are physical inactivity and excess body weight. Decreased gut motility, increased insulin resistance, lower metabolic rates, and increased circulating estrogens are all mechanisms implicated in the higher risk of colorectal cancer associated with this modifiable risk factor. [9, 10]

3.3. Modifiable risk factors: Social behaviors

Associated with a higher risk is regular consumption of cigarettes and alcohol. [10] Carcinogenic metabolites found in both tobacco and alcohol are considered promoters of tumor growth, based on experimental studies in animals. [15]

Cigarette-smoking has been attributed to 12% of colorectal cancer deaths, while alcohol consumption has been linked with early onset colorectal cancers, specifically tumors in the distal colon. [9, 16, 17] There is information showing that there is higher risk in active smokers for development of rectal cancer.[9, 18]

3.4. Nonmodifiable risk factors: Age

Increasing age carries a higher likelihood of colorectal cancer, specifically after the age of 40. [2]

Cancer incidence rises progressively after the age of 40 in the general population, with 90% of colorectal cancers occurring in those aged 50 years and older. [2] In fact, a 50-year old has 5% chance of developing cancer and 2.5% chance of dying from this cancer after the age of 80 years. [2, 9]

As such, the US Preventative Task Force (USPSTF) has defined "average risk" as those aged 50 years or more with no personal history of colorectal cancer or adenomas, no inflammatory bowel disease, and with negative family history. [19] Put in other terms, the incidence rate is more than 50 times higher in those 60–79 years old than in those less than 40 years old.

In contrast, those with "increased risk" include those with a personal history of colorectal cancer, personal history of colonic adenomas, family history of sporadic colorectal cancer, as well as family history of sporadic adenoma. [4, 9]

Finally, those with "high risk" include those with hereditary nonpolyposis colorectal cancer (Lynch syndrome), polyposis syndromes, and inflammatory bowel diseases (IBD). [4] *See below for a discussion on hereditary polyposis conditions and IBD.*

3.5. Nonmodifiable risk factors: Personal history of colonic adenomatous polyps

Carrying a personal history of adenomatous polyps has an increased risk of developing colorectal cancer, in comparison to those with no history of adenomas. In recent literature, it was reported that 95% of sporadic colorectal cancers developed from such adenomas, usually after a protracted period, which has been estimated anywhere from 5 to 10 years. [4, 9] However, while nearly all colorectal cancer arise from adenomas, only a small minority of these dysplastic polyps actually progress to cancer (5% or less). [4]

3.6. Nonmodifiable risk factors: Family history of colonic adenomatous polyps or colorectal cancer

The majority of cases occur in those with family history of either colorectal cancer or adenomatous cancer. In fact, there is a two- to three-fold increased risk of sporadic cancer in those with first-degree relatives. This means that up to 20% of those with colorectal cancer have family members affected by this disease. [4, 9] This risk becomes even higher when there are two or more relatives involved and when those family members are affected by the disease at an age younger than 60.

3.7. Nonmodifiable risk factors: Hereditary polyposis conditions

Those with recognized inherited polyposis syndromes carry an even higher risk. Recent literature estimates that about 5–10% of sporadic colorectal cancers are the outcome of inherited conditions, such as the familial adenomatous polyposis (FAP) and hereditary nonpolyposis colorectal cancer (HPNCC). [4, 9]

HPNCC (also called Lynch syndrome) is thought to comprise of about 1–6% of all colorectal cancers. It carries a lifetime risk of cancer as high as 70–80%. [4, 9] FAP and its variants account for less than 1% of all colorectal cancer cases, but almost all those diagnosed with this disorder will develop cancer if the colon is not removed by the age of 40. [4]

Other hereditary conditions that are associated with sporadic colorectal cancers include Gardner's syndrome (high-risk), Turcot's syndrome (high-risk), and Peutz-Jeghers syndrome (low-to-moderate risk). [4] Appropriate screening recommendations are made for this population subtype, which will not be discussed here.

3.8. Nonmodifiable risk factors: Personal history of Inflammatory Bowel Disease (IBD)

Those with IBD — ulcerative colitis and Crohn's disease — also carry an increased risk of developing colorectal cancer. It has been estimated that the relative risk of colorectal cancer in patients with IBD ranges from 4- to 20-fold. [4, 9] Thus, appropriate screening recommendations are made for this population subtype, which will not be discussed here.

4. Statistics

4.1. Methods

The following statistical data were obtained from the Surveillance, Epidemiology and End Results (SEER) Program of the National Cancer Institute (NCI), specifically from the data previously published in the *SEER Cancer Statistic Review (CSR) 1975–2012*, which was released in April 23, 2015. The NCI funds for the program through Centers for Disease Control and Presentation (CDC), National Program of Cancer Registries, and involved states' contributions.

The SEER program was conceptualized in 1973, with a mission to report the "most recent cancer incidence, mortality, survival, prevalence, and lifetime risks statistics. It originally only represented about 10% of the US population.

Since then, it has expanded to include the following population-based cancer registries: Alaska Native Tumor Registry, Arizona Indians, Cherokee Nation, Connecticut, Detroit, Georgia Center for Cancer Statistics (Atlanta, Greater Georgia, Rural Georgia), Greater Bay Area Cancer Registry (San Francisco-Oakland, San Jose-Monterey), Greater California, Hawaii, Iowa, Kentucky, Los Angeles, Louisiana, New Jersey, New Mexico, Seattle-Puget Sound, and Utah. This translates to approximately 26% of African Americans, 41% of Hispanics, 43% of American Indians and Alaska Natives, 54% of Asians, and 71% of Hawaiian/Pacific Islanders. It is published annually, with 2012 being the most recent year for which data are available.

4.2. Temporal trends in the united states

How common is this cancer? It is estimated that there will be 132,700 new colorectal cancer cases in 2015. [21] This comprises 8% of all new cancer cases (Figure 1). [21] Of those new cancer cases, there will be an estimated 49,700 deaths. [21] This comprises 8.4% of all cancer deaths (Table 4).

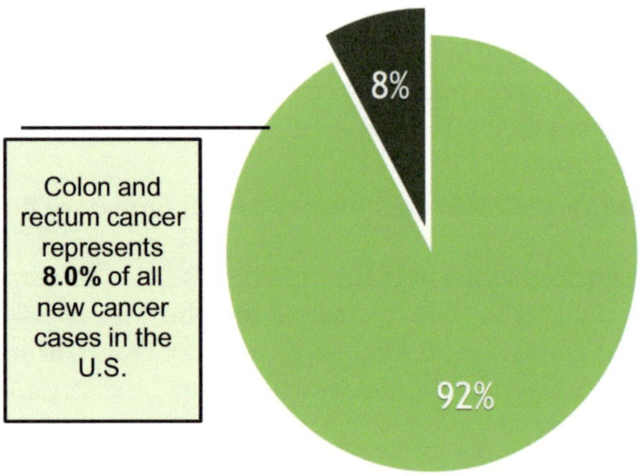

Figure 1. Colon and rectum cancer in the U.S.

Who gets this cancer? Colorectal cancer is more common in men than in women. In 2014, there were a total of 135,260 people diagnosed with colorectal cancer: 70,099 men versus 65,161 women. [22] Based on SEER 18, this means that 48.9 per 100,000 persons new cases were male, while 37.1 per 100,000 persons were female. [20]

Common Type of Cancer	Estimated New Cases 2015	Estimated Deaths 2015
Breast cancer (female)	231,840	40,290
Lung and bronchus cancer	221,200	158,040
Prostate cancer	220,800	27,540
Colon & rectal cancer	**132,700**	**49,700**
Bladder cancer	74,000	16,000
Melanoma of the skin	73,870	9,940
Non-Hodgkin Lymphoma	71,850	19,790
Thyroid cancer	62,450	1,950
Kidney & renal pelvis cancer	61,560	14,080
Endometrial cancer	54,870	10,170
Source: SEER 2015		

Table 4. Comparison of Common Cancers

While colorectal cancer is more common in men than in women, the gender bias is smaller when all races are included. However, the gender bias remains wide when race and ethnicity are factored in. The greatest divide was found in African American males versus females, with 61.2 per 100,000 new cases in black men versus 46.0 per 100,000 new cases in black women. [20]

Other race/ethnicities also showed a divide, but not as wide. Hispanic male new cases were 30/100,000 while female new cases were 43.3/100,000. American Indian/Alaska Native male new cases were 35.7/100,000 while female new cases were 46.3/100,000. Asian/Pacific Islander male new cases were 31.3/100,000 while female new cases were 42.2/100,000. White male new cases were 36.3/100,000 while female new cases were 47.8/100,000 (Table 5). [20]

At what age is this cancer most frequently diagnosed? Colorectal cancer is most frequently diagnosed among those aged 65–74 years old. [20] This age group comprises 23.9% of new cases. [20] The median age is 68 years old (Table 6; Figure 2).

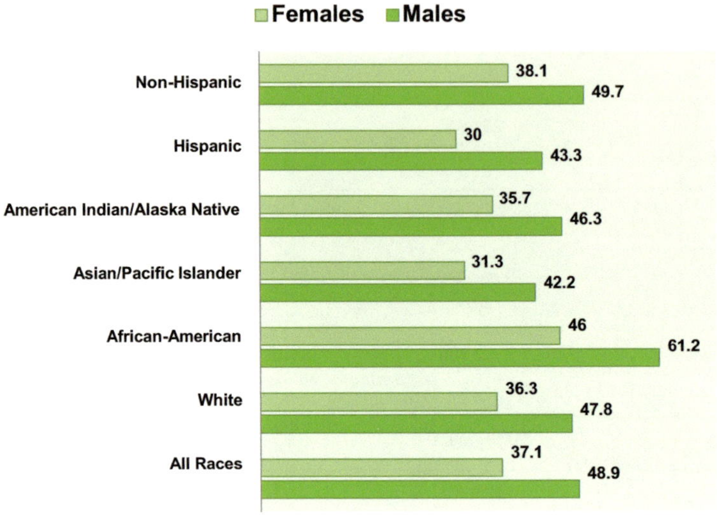

Source: SEER 18 2008-2012, Age Adjusted

Table 5. Number of New Colon and Rectal Cancer Cases/100,000 Persons by Race/Ethnicity & Sex

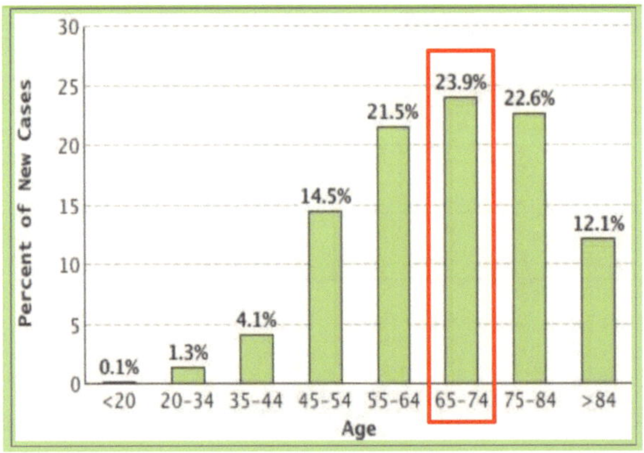

Source: SEER 2015

Table 6. Percent of Deaths by Age Group

There is different distribution based on age at diagnosis in different gender groups. In women, colon cancer tends to arise in an older population (mean age being 73 years old; Figure 2; in comparison, colon cancer tends to arise in a younger population in men (mean age being 69 years old; Figure 2). [9]

In the younger age groups (all races, both sexes), those <20 years old comprised of 0.1% of new cases; 20–34 years old comprised of 1.3%; 45–54 years old comprised of 14.5%; 55–64 years old comprised of 21.5%.

http://dx.doi.org/10.5772/61945

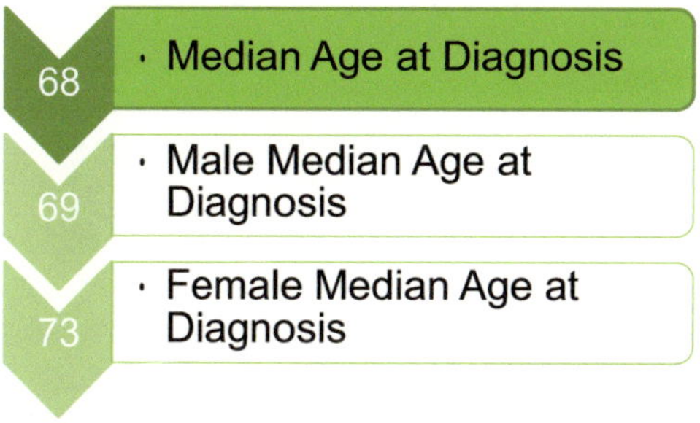

Figure 2. Median age at which colorectal cancer is most frequently diagnosed.

In the older age groups (all races, both sexes), 75–84 years old comprised of 22.6% (75–84 years old) and those >84 years old comprised of 12.1%. [20]

What are the survival rates? Based on the data from SEER 18 2005–2011, relative survival statistics show that 64.9% of people survive 5 years or more after being diagnosed with colon or rectal cancer (all races/sexes, Figure 3). [20, 22]

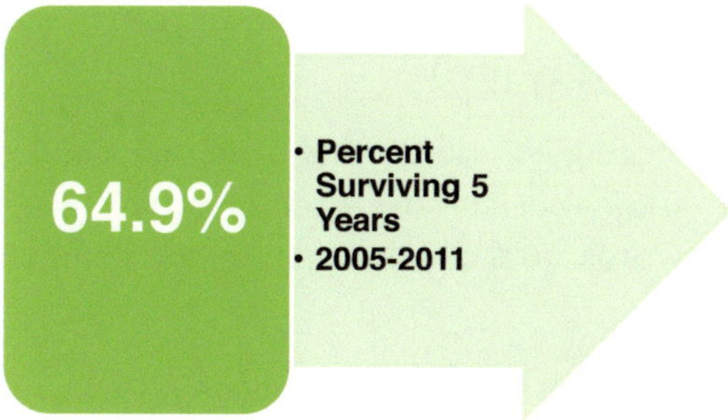

Figure 3. Relative survival rate of colon or rectal cancer.

Does staging influence survival rates? Cancer stage at diagnosis will determine both treatment options and has a strong influence on the length of survival. Obviously, the earlier the cancer is caught, the better the chance of survival.

Current statistics show that 39.5% of colon and rectal cancers are diagnosed at the local stage (confined to primary site), with a 5-year survival for localized colon and rectal cancer being very high at 90.1% [20] (Table 7).

Thirty-six percent of cancers in the regional stage (those spread to regional lymph nodes) have a 70.8% 5-year relative survival rate. [20] Twenty percent of cancers in the distant stage (those that metastasized) carry a 13.1% 5-year relative survival rate. [20] Lastly, those that are unstaged (5%) have a 34.5% 5-year survival rate [20] (Table 7).

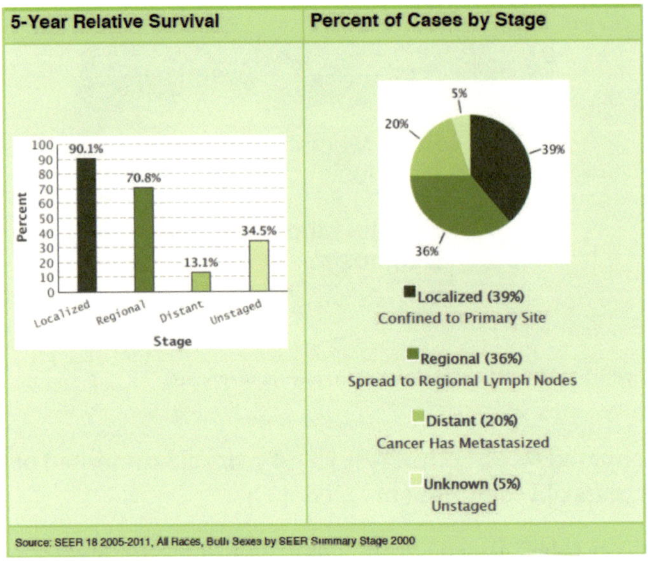

Table 7. 5-Year Relative Survival and Percent of Colon and Rectal Cancer Cases by Stage at Diagnosis [20]

Does the site of cancer change the incidence? Distribution of colon cancers also vary. This suggests that there are different pathogenic etiologies and carcinogenic mechanisms involved in different sites of the colon (and rectum).

The most common tumor locations in decreasing order are the descending colon (40–42%), rectosigmoid and rectum (30–33%), cecum and ascending colon (25–30%), and transverse colon (10–13%). [22, 23] In other words, 50% of colon cancers are within reach of a flexible sigmoidoscope [24] (Table 8).

Who dies from this cancer? As with all cancers, the death rates increase with age. Among both gender groups, it is the second leading cause of cancer deaths — behind lung cancer — with peak incidence being in the seventh decade of life. [2, 20]

In the United States, colorectal cancer is the second leading cause of death. [2] Unfortunately, each year there are >55,000 deaths (26,804 men; 24,979 women). [20]

The percent of deaths is highest among those aged 75–84 at 26.6%. [20] The median age at death is 73 years old (Figure 4). [20] This age group comprises 26.6% of all colorectal cancer deaths [20] (Table 9).

In the younger age groups (all races, both sexes), percent of deaths in those <20 years old comprised of 0% of new cases; 20–34 years old comprised of 0.7%; 35–44 years old comprised of 2.5%; 45–54 years old comprised of 9.3%; 55–64 years old comprised of 17.9%.

In the older age groups (all races, both sexes), percent of deaths in those 65–74 years old comprised of 22.1% and those >84 years old comprised of 21.0%. [20]

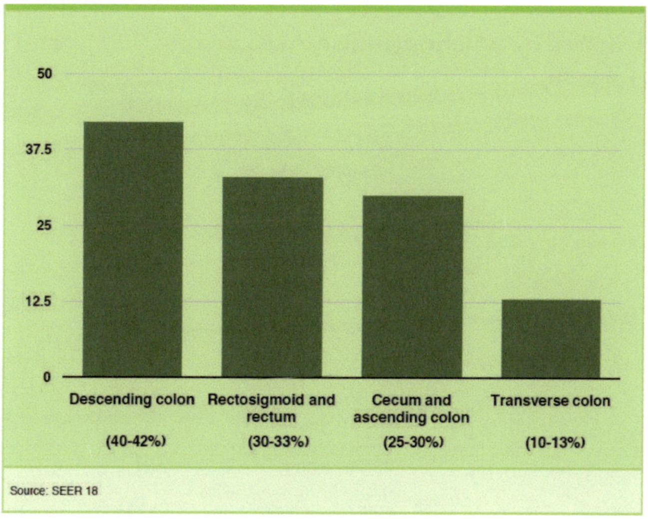

Table 8. Incidence Rates of Colon and Rectal Cancer by Location [20]

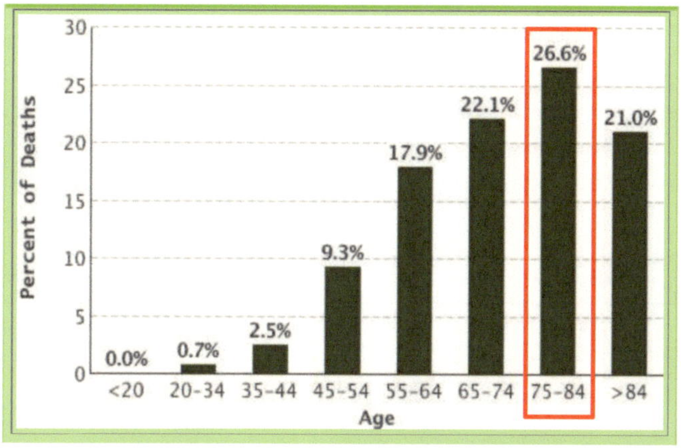

Source: SEER 18 2008-2012, All Races/Both Sexes

Table 9. Percent of Deaths by Age Group

As more males are diagnosed each year than females, there are more male number of deaths than females. In all races, there were 18.6 number of deaths per 100,000 males versus 13.1 number of deaths per 100,000 females.

The divide between the genders was even greater when race and ethnicity were factored in. African American males had the highest number of deaths per 100,000: 26.9 (versus 17.8/100,000 females). [25] Males who were identified as non-Hispanic (but not white or black) had the second highest number of deaths (18.9/100,000), followed by American Indian/Alaska native (18.8/100,000) and whites (18.0/100,000). Black females had the higher number of deaths per 100,000 (17.8), followed by American Indian/Alaska native (15.6), non-Hispanic (13.4), and whites (12.7) [20] (Table 10).

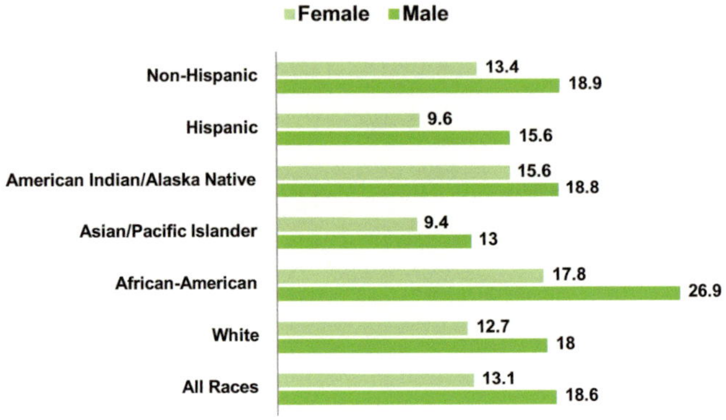

Source: U.S. 2008-2012, Age-Adjusted

Table 10. Number of Colon and Rectal Cancer Deaths per 100,000 Persons by Race/Ethnicity & Sex

What are the projection rates of colorectal cancer? Rates of new colon and rectal cancer diagnosis have been falling each year, over the past 10 years. [26] This is true not only for the United States but also for New Zealand, Australia, and Western Europe.[9] Despite these numbers, the death rate has not changed significantly, however (Table 11).

Year	1975	1980	1985	1990	1995	1999	2003	2007
5-Year Relative Survival	48.6%	51.1%	58.0%	60.8%	59.7%	64.5%	65.3%	66.5%

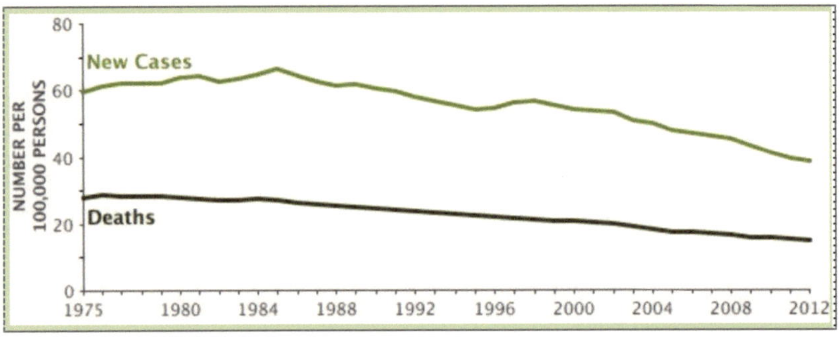

Source: SEER 9 Incidence & U.S. Mortality 1975-2012, all races/both sexes/rates are age-adjusted

Table 11. Incidence & U.S Mortality 1975-2012

5. Conclusion

Although new diagnosis rates of colorectal cancer have lowered significantly in both women and men since 1975, more can be done in terms of screening. The drama in these numbers is that colorectal cancer is a preventative cancer, both in screening and in identification of modifiable (i.e., theoretically preventable) risk factors. In fact, if everyone aged 50 years or older had regular screening tests, at least 60% of deaths from this cancer could have been avoided. [3, 19] And with the knowledge that the 5-year survival is close to 90% when colorectal cancer is diagnosed at an early stage, the statistics becomes even more dramatic. **Bottom-line:** colorectal cancer is susceptible to screening and aggressive campaigns toward educating the public dictate the future of its incidence and survival.

Author details

Camille Thélin* and Sanjay Sikka

*Address all correspondence to: cthelin1@tulane.edu

Department of Internal Medicine, Division of Gastroenterology and Hepatology, Tulane University, New Orleans, LA, United States

References

[1] Ferlay J, Soerjomataram I, Ervik M, Dikshit R, Eser S, Mathers C, Rebelo M, Parkin DM, Forman D, Bray, F. GLOBOCAN 2012 v1.1, Cancer Incidence and Mortality Worldwide: IARC CancerBase No. 11 [Internet]. Lyon, France: International Agency for Research on Cancer; 2014. Available from: http://www.wcrf.org/int/cancer-facts-figures/worldwide-data, accessed January 16, 2015.

[2] American Cancer Society, "Cancer Facts and Figures 2015." Reported by the North American Association of Central Cancer Registries (NAACCR). Available at http://www.cancer.org/acs/groups/content/@editorial/documents/document/acspc-044552.pdf.

[3] Centers for Disease Control and Prevention, Division of Cancer Prevention and Control. Colorectal Cancer Control Program (CRCCP) Fact Sheet. Available at cdc.gov/cancer/crccp/pdf/CRCCP_FactSheet.pdf, accessed December 2, 2013.

[4] Feldman M, Friedman LS, Brandt LJ. *Sleisenger and Fordtran's Gastrointestinal and Liver Disease: Pathophysiology, Diagnosis, Management, 10th Edition*. Philadelphia: Saunders/Elsevier, February 2010.

[5] Nawa T, Kato J, Kawamoto H, Okada H, Yamamoto H, Kohno H, Endo H, Shiratori Y. Differences between right- and left-sided colon cancer in patient characteristics, cancer morphology and histology. J Gastroenterol Hepatol 2008;23:418–23.

[6] American Cancer Society. Colorectal Cancer Facts and Figures 2014-2016. Atlanta: American Cancer Soceity, 2014. Available at http://www.cancer.org/acs/groups/content/documents/document/acspc-042280.pdf.

[7] Iacopetta B. Are there two sides to colorectal cancer? Int J Cancer 2002;101:403–8.

[8] Siegel RL, Jemal A, Ward EM. Increase in incidence of colorectal cancer among young men and women in the United States. Cancer Epidemiol Biomarkers Prev 2009;18:1695–8.

[9] Haggar FA, Boushey RP. Colorectal Cancer Epidemiology: Incidence, Mortality, Survival, and Risk Factors. Clinics in Colon and Rectal Surgery. 2009;22(4):191–7. doi: 10.1055/s-0029/1242458.

[10] Tárraga L, Pedro J, Albero JS, Rodríguez-Montes JA. "Primary and Secondary Prevention of Colorectal Cancer." Clinical Medicine Insights. Gastroenterology 2014;7:33–46. PMC. Web. 16 May 2015

[11] Doubeni CA, Laiyema AO, Major JM, et al. Socioeconomic status and the risk of colorectal cancer an analysis of more than a half million adults in the national Insittuaes of Health-AARP Diet and Health Study. Cancer 2012;118:3636–44.

[12] Boyle P, Langman JS. ABC of colorectal cancer: Epidemiology. BMJ 2000 Sept 30;321(7264):805–8.

[13] Santarelli R L, Pierre F, Corpet D E. Processed meat and colorectal cancer: a review of epidemiologic and experimental evidence. Nutr Cancer 2008;60(2):131–44

[14] Larsson S C, Wolk A. Meat consumption and risk of colorectal cancer: a meta-analysis of prospective studies. Int J Cancer 2006;119(11):2657–64

[15] Pöschl G, Seitz HK. Alcohol and cancer. Alcohol Alcohol 2004 May–Jun;39(3):155–65.

[16] Zisman AL, Nickolov A, Brand RE, Gorchow A, Roy HK. Associations between the age at diagnosis and location of colorectal cancer and the use of alcohol and tobacco: implications for screening. Arch Intern Med 2006;166(6):629–34.

[17] Botteri E, Iodice S, Raimondi S, Maisonneuve P, Lowenfels AB. Cigarette smoking and adenomatous polyps; a meta-analysis. Gastroenterology 2008;134(2);388–96; e3.

[18] Hooker CM, Gallicchio L, Genkinger JM, Comstock GW, Alberg AJ. A prospective cohort study of rectal cancer risk in relation to active cigarette smoking and passive smoke exposure. Ann Epidemiol 2008;18:28–35.

[19] US Preventative Task Force. Evaluating Test Strategies for Colorectal Cancer Screening: A Decision Analysis for the U.S. Preventive Services Task Force: Colorectal Cancer: Screening. November 2014. Available at http://

www.uspreventiveservicestaskforce.org/Page/SupportingDoc/colorectal-cancer-screening/evaluating-test-strategies-for-colorectal-cancer-screening-a-decision-analysis-for-the-us-preventive-services-task-force

[20] Howlader N, Noone AM, Krapcho M, Garshell J, Miller D, Altekruse SF, Kosary CL, Yu M, Ruhl J, Tatalovich Z,Mariotto A, Lewis DR, Chen HS, Feuer EJ, Cronin KA (eds). SEER Cancer Statistics Review, 1975-2012, National Cancer Institute. Bethesda, MD, http://seer.cancer.gov/csr/1975_2012/, based on November 2014 SEER data submission, posted to the SEER web site, April 2015

[21] U.S. Cancer Statistics Working Group. United States Cancer Statistics: 1999–2011 Incidence and Mortality Web-based Report. Atlanta: U.S. Department of Health and Human Services, Centers for Disease Control and Prevention and National Cancer Institute; 2014. www.cdc.gov/uscs.

[22] Siegel RL, Ward EM, Jemal A. Trends in colorectal cancer incidence rates in the United States by tumor location and stage, 1992-2008. Cancer Epidemiol Biomarkers Prev 2012;21:411–6.

[23] Seigel RL, DeSantis C, Jemal A. Colorectal cancer statistics, 2014. CA: Cancer J Clinicians 2014;64:104–17.

[24] Ferri F. *Ferri's Clinical Advisor 2015*, 1st ed. St. Louis, MO: Elsevier Mosby. 2014.

[25] American Cancer Society. Cancer facts & figures for African Americans 2005–2006. American Cancer Society, 2005. Available at http://www.cancer.org/docroot/STT/stt_0.asp, accessed November 8, 2005

[26] Chu KC, Tarone RE, Chow WH, Hankey BF, Ries LAG. Temporal patterns in colorectal cancer incidence, survival, and mortality from 1950 through 1990. J Natl Cancer Inst 1994;86:997–100.

Chapter 5

Basic Endoscopic Findings — Normal and Pathological Findings

Parth J. Parekh and Sanjay K. Sikka

Additional information is available at the end of the chapter

http://dx.doi.org/10.5772/61256

Abstract

Since its inception, colonoscopy has evolved to become the cornerstone for colorectal imaging. The increasing indications for endoscopic evaluation and potential therapeutic intervention parallels technological advances and the expanding diagnostic and therapeutic capabilities of colonoscopy. The diagnostic and therapeutic yield of colonoscopy is highly user dependent. Thus, it is essential for the clinical endoscopist to perform a thorough endoscopic evaluation and be cognizant of normal and pathologic findings. This review details normal and pathologic endoscopic findings in a variety of disease states that are often encountered by the clinical endoscopist including colon polyps, inflammatory bowel disease, and infectious and non-infectious colitides. In addition, we review the diagnostic and therapeutic role of colonoscopy in the evaluation of an acute lower gastrointestinal bleed.

Keywords: Polyp, pseudopolyp, hyperplastic polyp, adenoma, tubular adenoma, tubulovillous adenoma, sessile adenoma, sessile serrated adenoma, colitis, diverticulosis, hemorrhoids, anal fissure

1. Introduction

The advent of retrograde colonoscopy in June 1969 revolutionized the field of gastroenterology [1]. It has since evolved to become the gold standard for colorectal imaging [2, 3].

As technology continues to advance, so too does the diagnostic utility and therapeutic capabilities of colonoscopy. Thus, it becomes imperative for the clinical endoscopist to perform a thorough colonoscopic evaluation and be cognizant of normal and pathologic findings as indications for colonoscopy expand. Here, we detail normal and pathologic endoscopic findings in a variety of disease states that are often encountered by the clinical endoscopist including colon polyps, inflammatory bowel disease (IBD), and infectious and non-infectious colitides. In addition, we review the diagnostic and therapeutic role of colonoscopy in the evaluation of an acute lower gastrointestinal bleed.

2. Polyps and potential progression to colorectal cancer

Colorectal cancer is the third most common cancer among men and women, and the third leading cause of cancer-related death in the United States [4]. It is estimated that in 2014, 71,830 men and 65,000 women were diagnosed with colorectal cancer with approximately 50,000 mortalities (26,270 men and 24,040 women) as a result of the disease. Globally, colorectal cancer is the fourth leading cause of cancer-related death accounting for approximately 700,000 deaths in 2012 [5]. The vast majority of colorectal cancers stem from benign polyps arising from the mucosal layer. Winawer et al. were among the first to demonstrate that colorectal adenomas have the potential to progress to colorectal adenocarcinoma, thus stressing the importance of colonoscopic polypectomy in colorectal cancer prevention [6]. Subsequent long term data has validated the importance of colonoscopy and colonoscopic polypectomy in the prevention of colorectal cancer-related deaths [7]. To date, colonoscopy remains the cornerstone in colorectal cancer prevention. Unfortunately, the "miss rate" of colonoscopy for colorectal cancer and adenomas larger than 1 cm has been reported to be as high as 6% [8] and 17% [9, 10], respectively.

Adenomas and hamartomatous polyps, later discussed in depth, are polyps that carry malignant potential. They are indolent in nature, typically growing slowly over the span of a decade or more. There is a direct correlation between the size of the adenoma and its risk of developing future advanced adenomas or carcinoma with studies demonstrating this risk to be as high as 7.7% [11], 15.9% [11], and 19.3% [12], for adenomas <5mm, 5–20mm, and >20mm, respectively.

Chromosomal instability and common point mutations occurring in colorectal cancer-related tumor suppressor genes (e.g., APC, P53) or tumor promoter genes (e.g., K-Ras) architect the progression from benign polyps to colorectal cancer. Figure 1 depicts key point mutations and its impact on morphologic changes of a benign polyp to colorectal cancer. There is, however, considerable genetic and epigenetic heterogeneity resulting in different pathways to tumorigenesis [13]. Luo et al. sought to evaluate the effect of these alterations on the progression to colorectal cancer by conducting genome-wide array-based studies and comprehensive data analysis of aberrantly methylated loci in normal colon tissue (n=41), colon adenomas (n=42), and colorectal cancer (n=64) [14]. They identified three classes of cancers and two classes of adenomas, high-frequency methylation and low-frequency methylation based on their DNA methylation patterns. Mutant K-Ras was found in a subset of high-frequency methylated adenomas. In addition, they found the methylation signatures of high-frequency methylation adenomas to be similar to those of cancer with low or intermediate levels of methylation, and low-frequency methylation adenomas to have methylation signatures similar to that of normal colon tissue. These findings demonstrated genome-wide alterations in DNA methylation to

http://dx.doi.org/10.5772/61256

occur during the early stages of progression of adenomas to colorectal cancer, and the presence of heterogeneity in tumorigenesis, even at the adenoma step of the process.

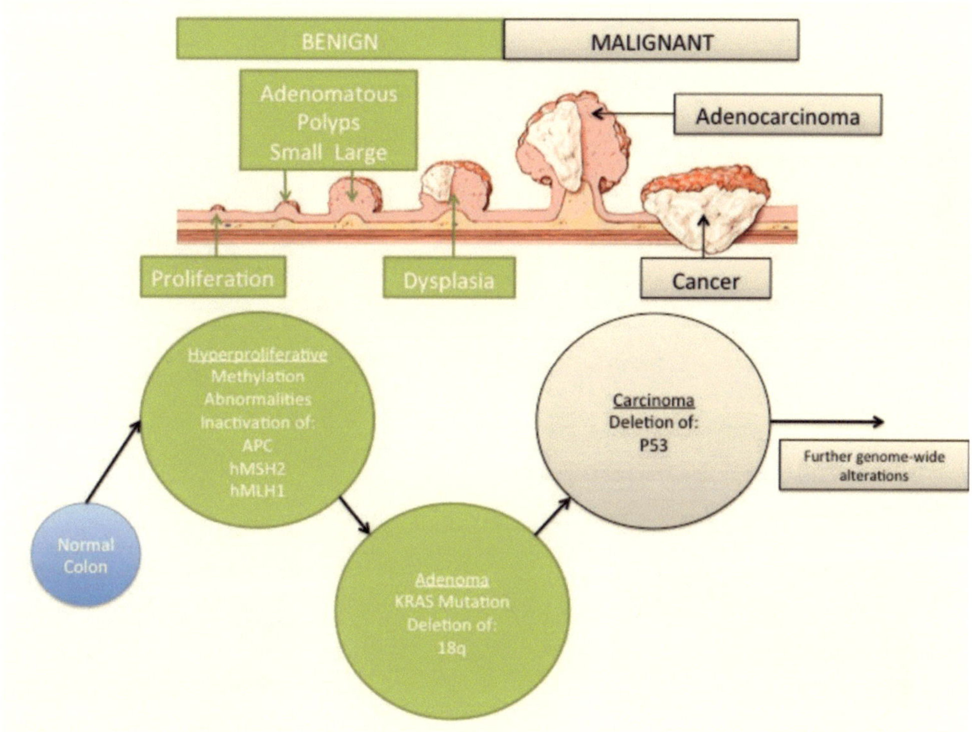

Figure 1. Key point mutations and its impact on morphologic changes of a benign polyp to colorectal cancer.

3. Polyps and pseudopolyps

In 2003, the Paris Endoscopic Classification arose to describe polyp morphology [15], which can potentially guide the endoscopist toward its malignancy potential [16–18]. Figure 2 provides a schematic overview of the Paris Endoscopic Classification and Figure 3 provides an endoscopic view of differing polyp morphology under traditional white-light colonoscopy. A recent study by van Doom et al. evaluated the interobserver agreement for the Paris Endoscopic Classification among seven expert endoscopists [19]. The seven expert endoscopists assessed 85 endoscopic video clips depicting polyps. Afterwards, they underwent a digital training module and then assessed the same 85 polyps again. A calculated Fleiss kappa of 0.42 and a mean pairwise agreement of 67% suggested moderate interobserver agreement among the seven experts. In addition, the proportion of lesions labeled as "flat" lesions ranged between 13–40% ($p<0.001$). The interobserver agreement did not change significantly after the digital training module, which led the investigators to conclude there to be only moderate interobserver agreement among experts for this classification system and that use of this classification system in daily practice is questionable and unsuitable for comparative endoscopist research. Thus, the need for a simplified classification system is necessary to better aid the clinical endoscopist.

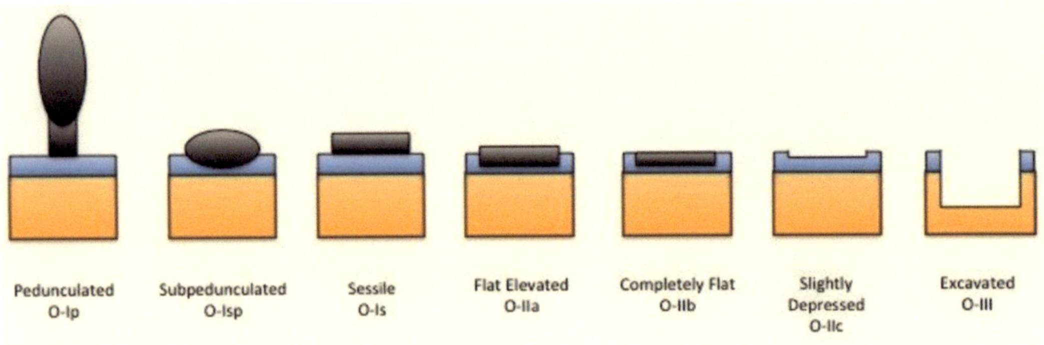

Figure 2. The Paris Classification based on polyp appearance.

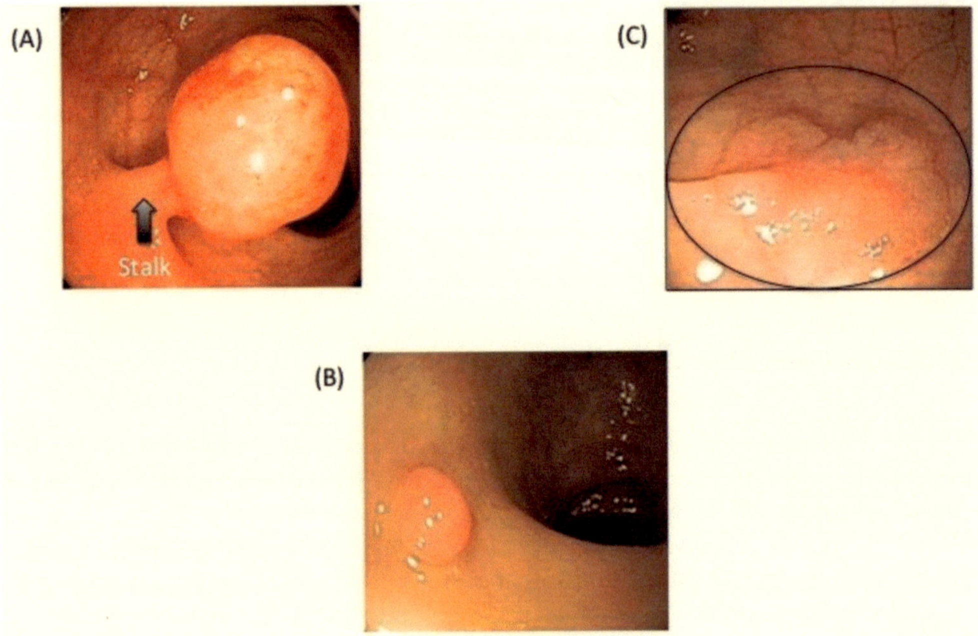

Figure 3. Endoscopic views of differing polyp morphology under traditional white-light colonoscopy: (A) Pedunculated polyp, (B) Sessile polyp, (C) Flat polyp.

In addition to traditional white-light colonoscopy, several studies have demonstrated the utility of narrow-band-imaging (NBI) to be useful in adenoma detection [20–23]. Under NBI, adenomas appear to have thicker and higher volumes of microvasculature compared to normal mucosa and hyperplastic polyps, resulting in distinct pit patterns that may increase diagnostic yield [23]. This section will review the morphology and histology, malignant potential, and provide endoscopic and pathologic depictions of different polyp subtypes.

3.1. Adenomas

Adenomatous polyps by definition are dysplastic and thus carry malignant potential. They can further be characterized as being an advanced adenoma, synchronous adenoma, or metachronous adenoma. An advanced adenoma is defined as an adenoma with high-grade dysplasia, an adenoma with a size >10 mm, an adenoma with significant villous components (>25%), or an adenoma with evidence of invasive carcinoma [24]. Synchronous adenomas are polyps that are diagnosed at the same time as an index colorectal cancer and metachranous adenomas are ones diagnosed at least six months before or after the diagnosis of an index colorectal cancer [25]. The diagnosis of synchronous and metachranous adenomas are of utmost importance as it can potentially identify individuals at risk for hereditary conditions, thus impacting therapeutic intervention and screening intervals for relatives [26].

3.1.1. Tubular, villous, and tubulovillous adenomas

Adenomas are characterized as tubular, villous, or tubulovillous (a mixture of the two) based on their glandular architecture. Tubular adenomas, which account for the vast majority of colon adenomas, are characterized by a network of branching adenomatous epithelium and a tubular component of >75% [16]. Figure 4 depicts a histologic representation of a tubular adenoma in the background of normal colon tissue. Villous adenomas, which account for up to 15% of adenomas, are characterized by long glands that extend straight down to the center of the polyp from its surface with a villous component of >75% [16]. Figure 5 depicts a histologic representation of a villous adenoma in the background of normal colon tissue. Lastly, tubulovillous adenomas, which account for up to 15% of adenomas, are a mixture of the two previous adenomas with a villous component of anywhere from 26–75%. Figure 6 depicts a histologic representation of a tubulovillous adenoma in the background of normal colon tissue.

The CpG island methylator phenotype (CIMP) pathway is composed of methylated promoter regions of multiple putative tumor suppressor genes occurring in colorectal cancer and also in adenomatous polyps [27]. Kakar et al. examined villous/tubulovillous adenomas (n=32) and tubular adenomas (n=30) for *BRAF*/K-Ras mutations and CIMP-status (characterized by methylation of three or more loci at hMLH1, p16, HIC1, RASSF2, MGMT, MINT1, and MINT31) [28]. They found 44% of villous/tubulovillous to be CIMP-positive compared with 27% of tubular adenomas (p=0.08). In addition, villous/tubulovillous adenomas demonstrated significantly higher methylation rates at MGMT (87% vs. 37%; p<0.01) and RASSF2 (94% vs. 70%; p=0.02) when compared to tubular adenomas. Lastly, CIMP-positive adenomas correlated with increased size, right-sided location, and increased villous component in villous/tubulovillous adenomas. This led the authors to conclude that CIMP status is indicative of size, location, and malignant potential, and that methylation of MGMT and RASSF2 increases as adenomas progress from tubular adenomas to villous/tubulovillous adenomas.

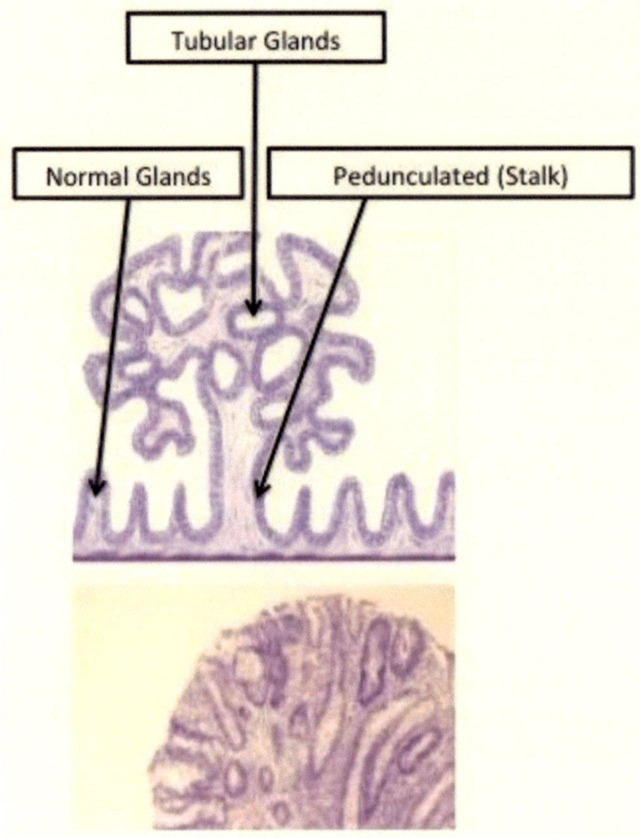

Figure 4. Histologic representation of tubular adenoma in the background of normal colon tissue.

3.1.2. Sessile serrated adenomas, traditional serrated adenomas, and hyperplastic polyps

Serrated lesions account for approximately 30% of colorectal cancers, arising via the serrated neoplasia pathway characterized by widespread DNA methylation and *BRAF* mutations [29]. They are classified histologically as sessile serrated adenomas/polyps (SSA/Ps), traditional serrated adenomas (TSAs), or hyperplastic polyps, with only SSA/Ps and TSAs carrying malignant potential [30]. SSA/Ps typically lack classic dysplasia, however, those that demonstrate foci of classic histologic dysplasia and molecular profiles exhibiting methylation of DNA repair genes (e.g., MLH-1) are thought to be precursor lesions to sporadic unstable microsatellite (MSI-H) cancers. SSA/Ps also exhibit activation of the *BRAF* oncogene, a feature seen in many sporadic MSI-H cancers [31]. Figure 7 depicts two potential molecular pathways of serrated neoplasia.

SSA/Ps tend to be more prominent in the proximal colon [32] as compared with TSAs [33] and hyperplastic polyps [34], which tend to be more prominent in the rectosigmoid. Thus, expert recommendations are to completely remove all serrated lesions proximal to the sigmoid colon and all serrated lesions in the rectosigmoid >5mm [30]. They may be more difficult to detect

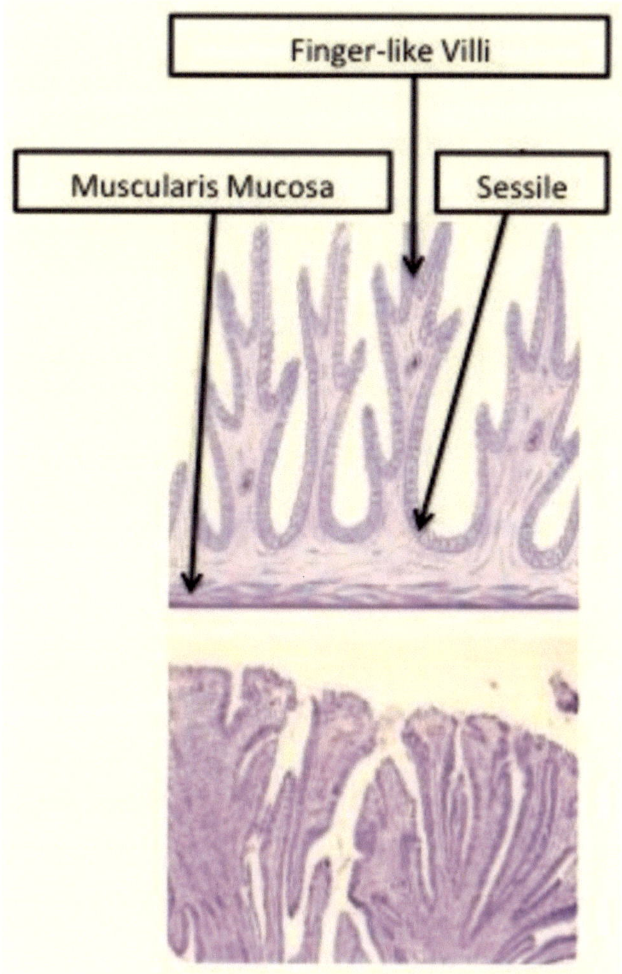

Figure 5. Histologic representation of villous adenoma in the background of normal colon tissue.

than conventional adenomatous polyps, in particular SSA/Ps, since they are more likely to be flat lesions, and so recent studies have advocated for a longer withdrawal time to increase serrated lesion detection rates [35, 36].

Serrated lesions have a distinct endoscopic appearance albeit often very subtle. A retrospective analysis of high-resolution endoscopic video clips by Tadepalli et al. analyzed the gross morphologic characteristics of 158 SSPs [37]. They found the most prevalent visual descriptors to be the presence of a mucous cap (which may be yellow or green in white light and red under NBI) (63.9%), rim of debris or bubbles (51.9%), alteration of the contour of a fold (37.3%), and interruption of underlying vascular pattern (32%). Figure 8 depicts an SSP under traditional white-light colonoscopy with a superficial mucous cap, its appearance under NBI, and a histologic representation.

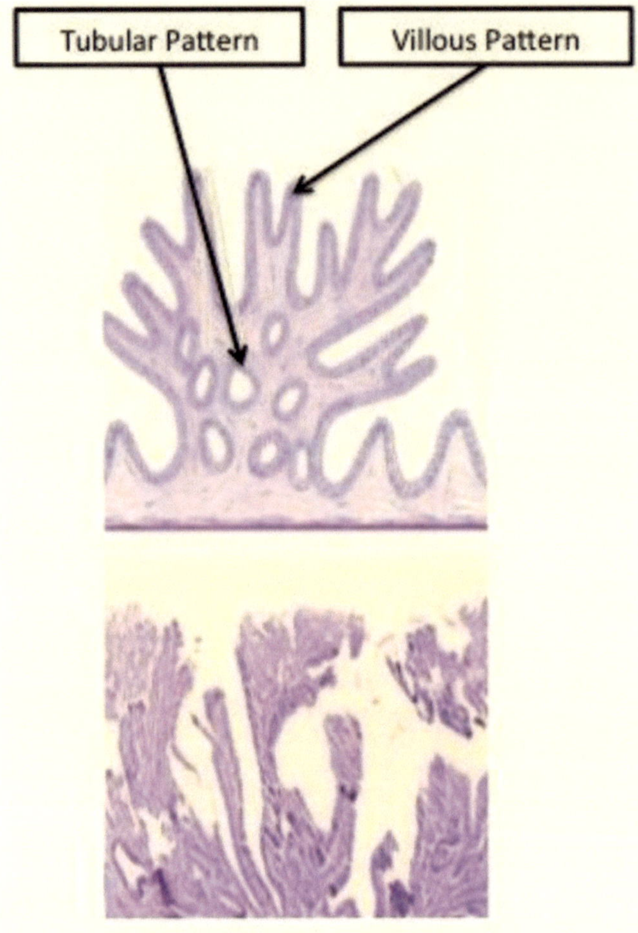

Figure 6. Histologic representation of a tubulovillous adenoma in the background of normal colon tissue.

Hyperplastic polyps are the most common non-neoplastic polyps in the colon; however, they are oftentimes grossly indistinguishable from adenomatous polyps. Histologically, hyperplastic polyps resemble normal colonic tissue with the exception of proliferation in the basal portion of the crypt and a characteristic "saw tooth" pattern along the crypt axis [38]. The relationship between diminutive hyperplastic polyps in the left colon and proximal neoplasia has long been a topic of debate with studies producing mixed results [39–42]. Hyperplastic polyps found proximal to the left colon, however, have consistently been shown to carry malignant potential and should be resected [39, 43].

3.2. Hamartomatous polyps

Hamartomatous polyps are polyps that may grossly resemble normal colonic tissue but are histologically a mixture of tissues growing in disarray. Histologically, they contain mucous-filled glands, retention cysts, abundant connective tissue, and/or chronic eosinophilic infiltra-

http://dx.doi.org/10.5772/61256

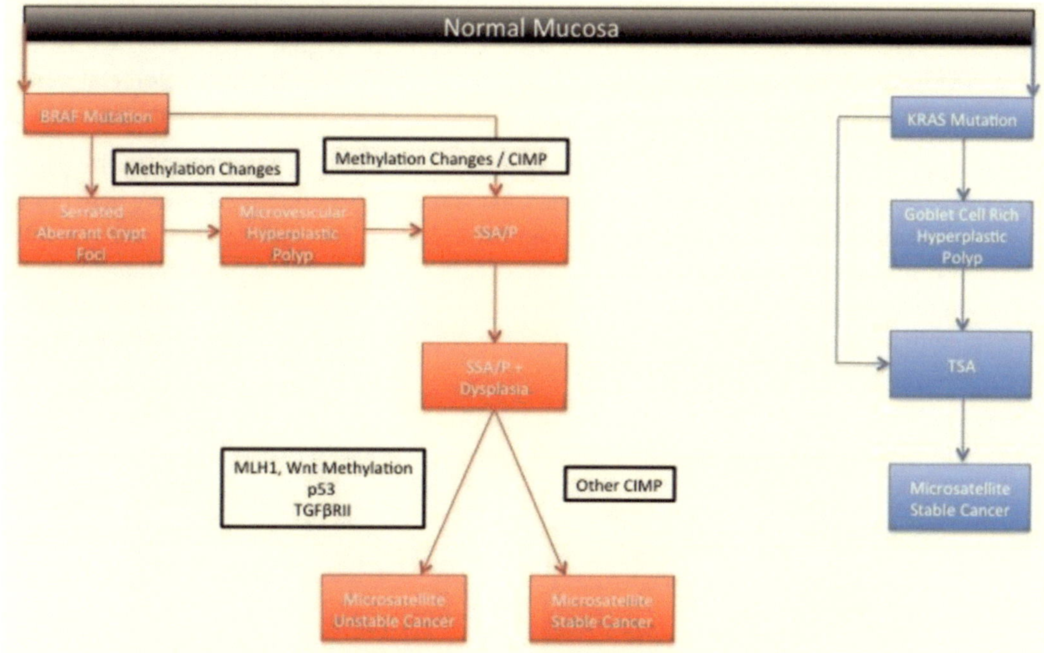

Figure 7. Potential molecular pathways of serrated neoplasia.

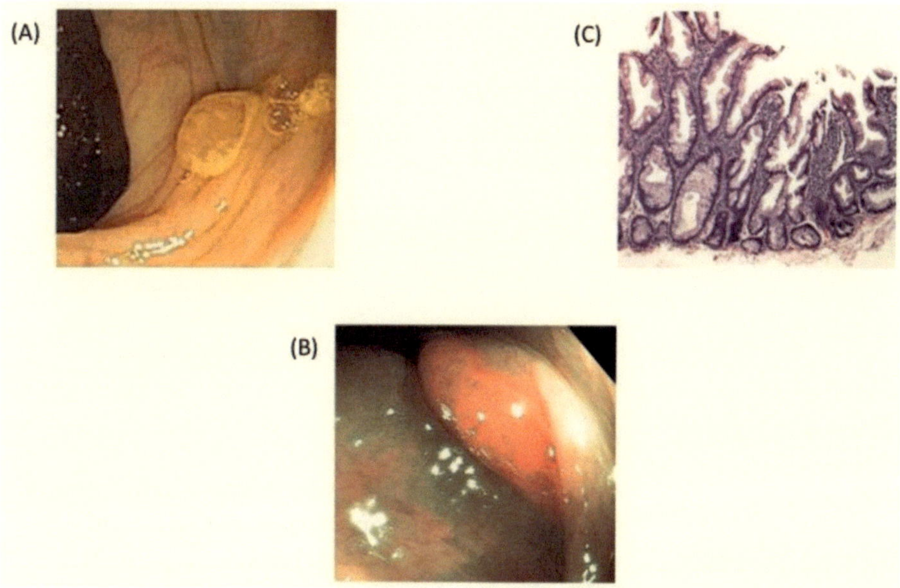

Figure 8. A) Sessile serrated polyp with mucosal cap under white-light colonoscopy. (B) Sessile serrated polyp under NBI. (C) Histology of sessile serrated polyp demonstrating expanded crypt proliferative zone, exaggerated architecture in crypt region with basilar crypt dilation, inverted crypts, and a predominance of crypts with minimal cell maturation.

tion [44]. Traditionally, they have been classified as non-neoplastic but several associated polyposis syndromes (e.g., Juvenile Polyposis Coli, Peutz-Jegher Syndrome, Cronkhite Canada Syndrome, and Cowden Syndrome) do carry a predilection towards colorectal cancer and other gastrointestinal malignancies.

Juvenile polyps are a type of hamartomatous polyp characterized by dilated cystic glands rather than an increased number of epithelial cells [44]. They can be found at any age, but as the name implies, are more commonly diagnosed during childhood. They are typically removed due to their propensity to bleed. Peutz-Jegher polyps are a type of hamartomatous polyp characterized by glandular epithelium supported by smooth muscle cells contiguous with the muscularis mucosa. Figure 9 depicts an endoscopic view of a hamartomatous polyp and histologic view of a Peutz-Jegher polyp.

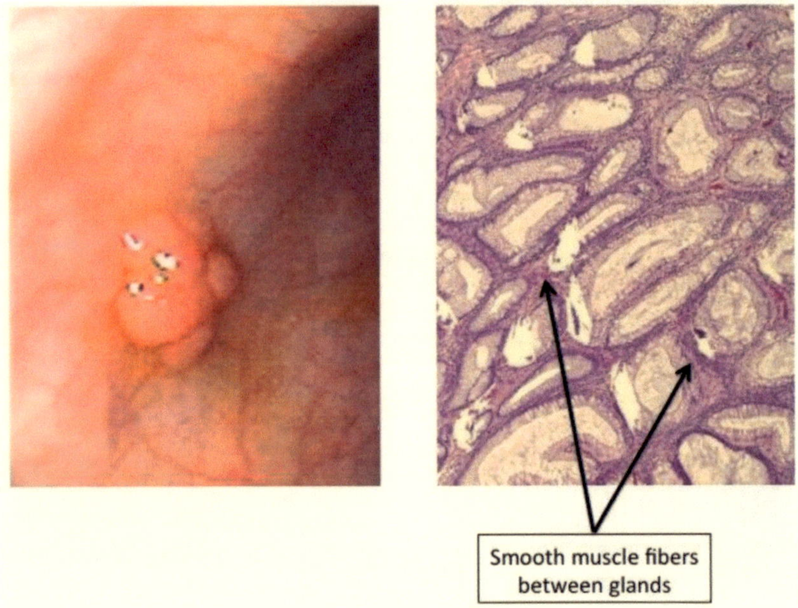

Figure 9. Endoscopic view of a hamartomatous polyp and histologic view of a Peutz-Jegher polyp.

3.3. Inflammatory pseudopolyps

Inflammatory polyps, typically seen in IBD, are indicative of regenerative and/or healing phases of mucosal ulceration and possess no malignant potential. They are formed from discrete islands of residual intact colonic mucosa that result from the ulceration and tissue regeration that is inherent to the disease course [45]. Scattered throughout the colitic region of the colon, they are often numerous, filiform, and can be large enough to encompass the lumen resulting in intussusception or luminal obstruction [45, 46]. The clinical endoscopist ought to be cognizant of clusters of localized giant pseudopolyposis as they may be associated with occult dysplasia [47]. Histologically, inflammatory pseudopolyps are characterized by

http://dx.doi.org/10.5772/61256

inflamed lamina propria and distorted colonic epithelium [48]. Surface erosions, congestion, hemorrhage and/or crypt abscesses may also be present [48]. Figure 10 depicts an endoscopic and histologic view of an inflammatory pseudopolyp.

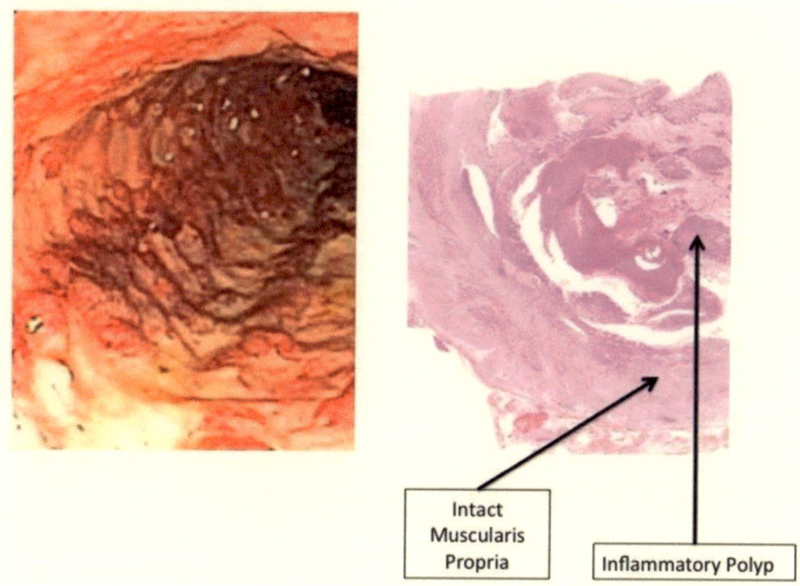

Figure 10. Endoscopic and histologic view of an inflammatory pseudopolyp.

4. Colitis

4.1. Inflammatory bowel disease

In patients with a clinical presentation suggestive of IBD, colonoscopy with ileoscopy can be used to make the initial diagnosis as it allows for direct visualization and biopsy of rectal, colonic, and terminal ileum mucosa [49]. In addition, it can assess disease activity and monitor therapeutic response, provide surveillance of dysplasia or neoplasia, and lastly provide therapeutic intervention such as stricture dilation [49] or closure of fistulae and anastomotic leakages [50].

The use of endoscopic appearance in distinguishing IBD from other non-IBD colitides is limited [51] as there are a number of 'IBD mimickers' including but not limited to colonic tuberculosis [52], Behçet's disease [53], and segmental colitis associated with diverticular disease [54]. In addition to tuberculosis, there are hosts of other infectious colitides that can also endoscopically mimic IBD [51, 55]. Table 1 provides an endoscopic description of various infectious colitides. Once these other etiologies have been excluded, colonoscopy can often shed light in distinguishing Crohn's disease (CD) from ulcerative colitis (UC), which is important for disease management. The data gathered from an index colonoscopy is of utmost importance owning to the fact that once therapy is initiated for IBD, discriminating features of CD from UC may be obscured [56, 57].

Infectious Etiology	Endoscopic Appearance
Apergillus	Hemorrhagic ulcerations
Campylobacter	Colonic erythema and ulceration
Chlamydia	Perianal abscesses, ulcerations, and fistulae
C. difficile	Pseudomembranes and moderately severe colitis, predominantly left sided
Cytomegalovirus	Colitis with ulceration (typically punched out and shallow)
Entamoeba	Acute colitis with ulceration
E. coli 0157:H7	Moderately severe colitis
Herpes	Proctitis with ulceration, there may be perianal involvement as well.
Histoplasma	Moderately severely colitis, predominantly right sided
Klebsiella	Hemorrhagic colitis
Mycobacterium	Ileal ulceration, may be transverse or circumferential
Nessieria	Proctitis with ulceration, there may be perianal involvement as well
Salmonella	Friable mucosa, ileal and colonic hemorrhages often present
Schistosoma	Extensive colitis may be segmental, polyps often times present
Shigella	Intense patchy colonic erythema that can also include the ileum
Treponema	Proctitis with ulceration, there may be perianal involvement as well
Yersinia	Patchy colitis with ileal ulceration (apthoid)

Table 1. Endoscopic description of various infectious colitides [54].

4.1.1. *Endoscopic features of UC and Mayo Scoring System*

Endoscopically, classic UC starts in the rectum and progresses proximally, sometimes as far as the ileo-cecal valve, in a circumferential and contiguous fashion with diffused and continuous inflammation [58]. Endoscopic features suggestive of UC include erythema, edema resulting in a loss of the usual vascular patter, granular appearing mucosa, increased friability, and small superficial erosions and ulcers surrounded by diffuse inflammation [59]. These classic visual features are used to endoscopically score the extent of the disease. The Mayo

http://dx.doi.org/10.5772/61256

Scoring System was derived in order provide an objective measure describing the endoscopic extent of the disease. Lemmens et al. sought to evaluate the correlation between endoscsopy and histology with use of the Mayo Scoring System [60]. This retrospective study included 236 biopsy sets from 131 patients with known UC. Endoscopy was performed by IBD specialists and graded using the Mayo Scoring System. Biopsy specimens were analyzed by expert gastrointestinal pathologists using the Geboes and Riley histologic scoring systems. They found that at both extremes, inactive and severely active disease, there was a very high concordance rate. For mild disease, however, there were important differences, as histologic examination seemed to have detected more severe disease than endoscopically suspected, thus stressing the need for a combined histologic and endoscopic scoring system when assessing disease activity. Figure 11 depicts the classic endoscopic appearance of UC in relation to the Mayo Scoring System.

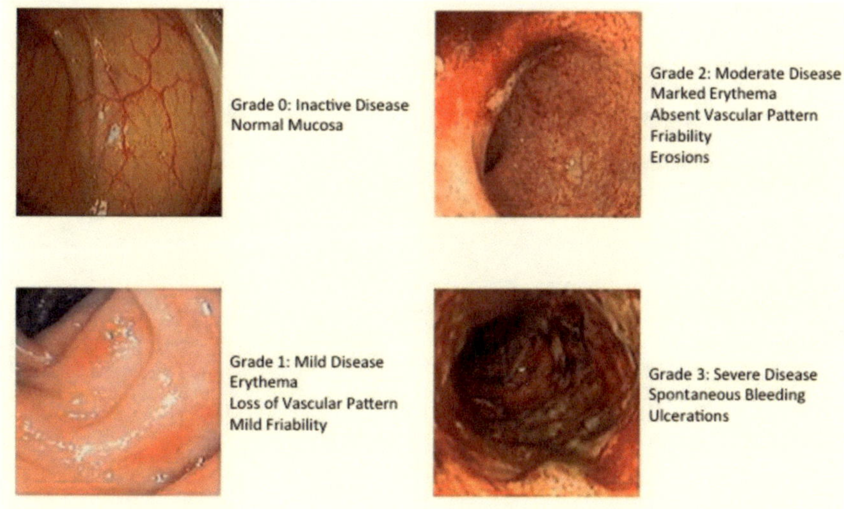

Figure 11. Classic endoscopic appearance of UC in relation to the Mayo Scoring System.

4.1.2. *Endoscopic features of CD and the Simple Endoscopic Score for CD (SES-CD)*

Inflammation in CD can span the entire gastrointestinal tract with nearly 55% of cases involving the terminal ileum and colon, 40% involving exclusively the ileum, and 25% involving the colon alone [61]. Rectal involvement occurs in up to 50% of patients with CD [62]. It should be noted that while terminal ileal involvement is strongly suggestive of CD, it might also occur in patients with UC, particularly pan-colitic UC, by way of "backwash" of cecal contents or "backwash ileitis" [63, 64]. The exact pathogenesis of "backwash ileitis" remains poorly understood, however it is believed that in patients with pan-colitic UC, the terminal ileum becomes inflamed stemming from chronic exposure to cecal contents.

Endoscopically, classic CD appears as "skip lesions" or areas of inflammation interposed between islands of normal mucosa, "cobblestone" appearance of the mucosal surface due to submucosal inflammation and edema, and deep, longitudinal, polycyclic ulcers [55]. In 2004, the SES-CD was derived in order to provide an objective measure describing the endoscopic extent of the disease [65]. To date, prospective data evaluating the utility of SES-CD in predicting corticosteroid-free clinical remission and long-term disease progression is lacking [66, 67]. Figure 12 depicts the classic endoscopic appearance of CD as well as the SES-CD. Table 2 illustrates the key endoscopic differences between UC and CD.

	SES-Score			
Variable	0	1	2	3
Size of ulcer (diameter in cm)	None	Aphthous ulcers (0.1-0.5)	Large ulcers (0.5-2)	Very large ulcers (>2)
Ulcerated surface (%)	None	<10	10-30	>30
Affected surface (%)	Unaffected segment	<50	50-75	>75
Presence of strictures	None	Single, can be passed	Multiple, can be passed	Cannot be passed

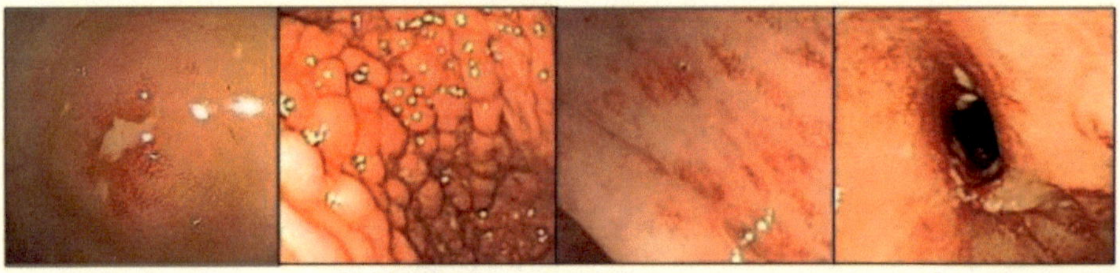

Figure 12. Classic endoscopic appearance of CD as well as the SES-CD.

Endoscopic Features	Ulcerative Colitis	Crohn's Disease
Aphthous Ulcers	√	√√√
Cobblestone Appearance	x	√√
Deep Ulcers	x	√√√
Erythema	√√√	√√
Granular Mucosa	√√√	√
Ileal Ulcers	x	√√√
Loss of Vascular Pattern	√√√	√
Pseudopolyp	√√√	√√√
Patchy Inflammation	x	√√√
Rectal Involvement	√√√√	√√

Table 2. Key endoscopic differences between UC and CD [54].

http://dx.doi.org/10.5772/61256

4.2. Microscopic (Lymphocytic and collagenous) and eosinophilic colitis

While microscopic colitis by definition is a histologic diagnosis, emerging data suggests that it may not always present with normal endoscopic findings [68–72]. Microscopic colitis is further subdivided into lymphocytic colitis and collagenous colitis depending on the presence of lymphocytic predominant infiltration or collagen deposition, respectively [73]. There have been several macroscopic lesions associated with collagenous colitis including longitudinal ulcers [69,70], hypervascularity [71], loss of normal vascularity [72], and exudative bleeding [73]. A retrospective study by Park et al. sought to investigate macroscopic lesions seen on the endoscopy in 14 patients with diagnosed lymphocytic colitis [68]. Patients with more severe diarrhea demonstrated macroscopic lesions on colonoscopy that included hypervascularity and exudative bleeding, which led to the conclusion that lymphocytic colitis may not always present with a normal endoscopically appearing mucosa. Figure 13 depicts lymphocytic colitis associated with hypervascular mucosa and exudative bleeding.

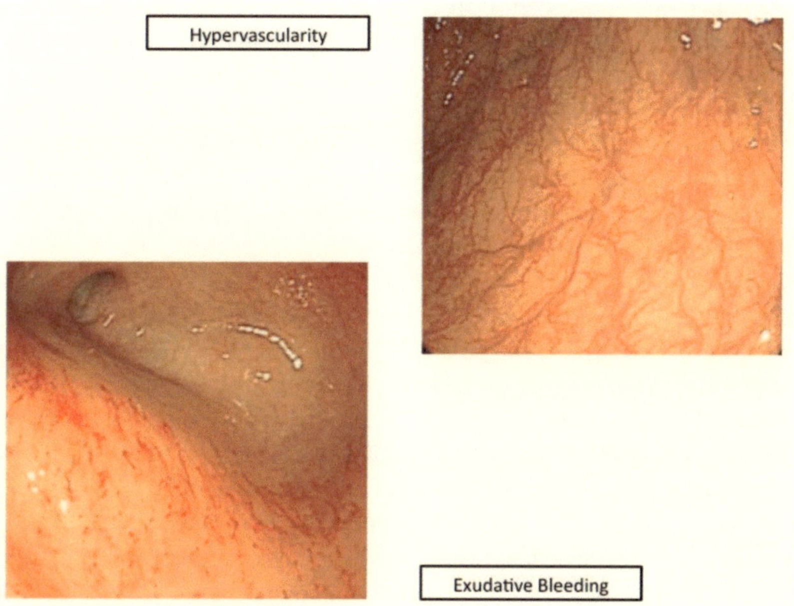

Figure 13. Hypervascular mucosa and exudative bleeding associated with lymphocytic colitis.

Eosinophilic disorders can span the entirety of the gastrointestinal tract, including the esophagus (eosinophilic esophagitis), stomach and small intestine (eosinophilic gastroenteritis), and the colon (eosinophilic colitis). Eosinophilic colitis is the least frequent manifestation of primary eosinophilic gastrointestinal disorders with only a few reports reported over the last four decades [74]. Secondary eosinophilic colitis can stem from several conditions including parasitic infections (e.g., *Strongyloides stercoralis* [75], *Enterobius vermicularis* [76], and *Trichuris trichiura* [77]), drug-induced (e.g., clozapine [78], carbamazepine [79], rifampicin [80], non-steroidal anti-inflammatory drugs [81, 82], tacrolimius [83], and gold [84]), auto-immune disorders (e.g., scleroderma [85], dermatomyositis and polymyositis [86, 87], and vasculitides (e.g., Churg-Strauss syndrome [88]). Endoscopic features suggestive of eosinophilic colitis include an edematous mucosa with loss of normal vascular pattern, patchy erythema, and superficial ulcerations [74].

4.3. Ischemic colitis

Ischemic colitis occurs as a result of inadequate blood supply to the large colon, typically affecting the critically ill and elderly population [89]. A recent retrospective study by Church et al. examined the role of urgent bedside colonoscopy in critically ill patients [90]. This study included 41 patients totaling 49 bedside colonoscopies with the most common indication being to exclude ischemic colitis (n=25). Of those 25, the diagnosis was confirmed in 19 with 14 patients subsequently undergoing surgical intervention, which led the authors to conclude that bedside colonoscopy is helpful in the diagnosis of acute lower gastrointestinal disease and can potentially guide therapeutic management in critically ill patients. There are several endoscopic findings that may assist in the diagnosis of ischemic colitis, one of which is the colon single-stripe sign. Zuckerman retrospectively studied 26 patients with endoscopic evidence of the colon single-stripe sign and compared it with 58 consecutive patients without a stripe [91]. All patients in the colon single-strip cohort had a stripe that was >5cm in length predominantly in the left colon (89%). Patients with the colon single-stripe sign were significantly more likely to have evidence of a preceding ischemic event (62%) compared to the colitis comparison group (7%). Histologically, patients with the colon single-stripe sign had microscopic evidence of ischemic injury compared to the colitis cohort (75% vs. 13%, respectively; $p<0.0001$). Next, the clinical course and outcome of the 26 patients with the colon single-stripe sign was compared with 22 patients with circumferentially involved ischemic colitis. None of the patients with the colon single-stripe sign required surgical intervention compared with 27% of patients with circumferential ischemic colitis. In addition, mortality rates were higher in the circumferential ischemic colitis group compared with patients with the colon single-stripe sign (41% vs. 4%, respectively; $p<0.05$). This led the authors to conclude that the colon-single stripe sign can manifest endoscopically, typically in a milder disease in the clinical spectrum of ischemic colitis [91]. Other endoscopic manifestations of ischemic colitis include petechial hemorrhages, edematous and fragile mucosa, segmental erythema, scattered erosions, and longitudinal ulcerations [92]. The 'watershed areas' areas (e.g., splenic flexure and transverse colon) are areas most vulnerable to ischemia due to the fact that they have the fewest collateral circulation. Figure 14 depicts various endoscopic manifestations of ischemic colitis.

4.4. Graft-Versus-Host Disease (GVHD)

Acute GVHD is associated with significant morbidity and mortality in the first 100 days following allogeneic hematopoietic progenitor stem cell transplant [93]. Acute GVHD can have GI manifestations (abdominal pain, nausea/vomiting, and diarrhea), obstructive jaundice, or skin rash. Gastroenterologists are often times consulted for endoscopic evaluation to rule out GHVD, when post-transplant patients present with GI manifestations in the absence of liver

http://dx.doi.org/10.5772/61256

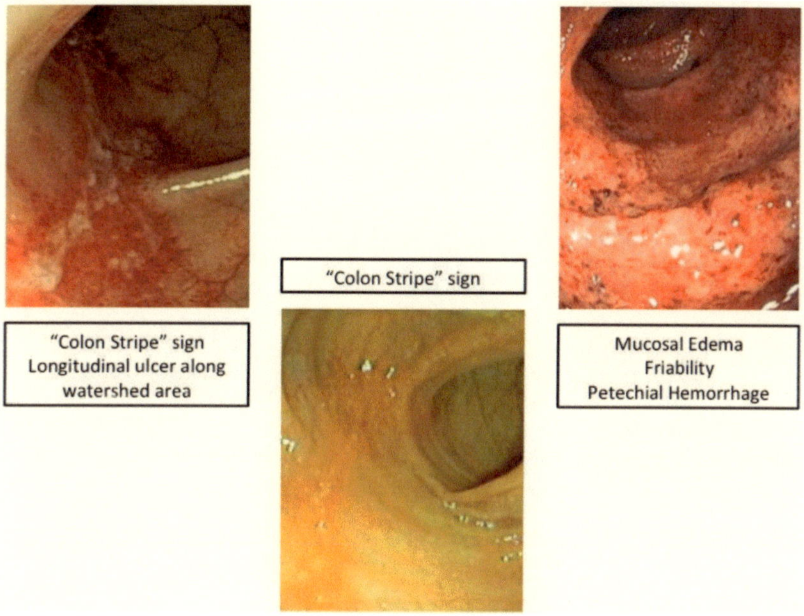

Figure 14. Various endoscopic manifestations of ischemic colitis.

or dermatologic involvement. In a majority of patients, flexible sigmoidoscopy with rectal biopsies allow for histologic diagnosis of GVHD and thus colonoscopy is not necessary [94, 95]. Endoscopic features of GVHD include diffuse edema, hyperemia, patchy erosions, scattered ulcers, sloughing, and active bleeding [96].

5. Evaluation of Lower Gastrointestinal Bleeding (LGIB)

The incidence of LGIB is approximately 20 per 100,000, with an associated all cause mortality of 3.9% [97]. The three most common causes of LGIB include angioectasias, diverticular bleeding, and hemorrhoidal bleeding [98]. Colonic ulcerations secondary to underlying IBD or chronic NSAID use, stercoral ulcer, Dieulafoy's lesion, or colorectal varices are less common etiologies of LGIB. In addition, an upper gastrointestinal source should also be included in the differential being that upwards of 15% of patients with severe hematochezia are found to have an upper gastrointestinal source [99]. In a hemodynamically stable patient, colonoscopy remains the cornerstone in the diagnosis of an LGIB. Figure 15 is a suggested algorithm by Parekh et al. for the role of colonoscopy in the evaluation of a hemodynamically stable LGIB [100].

Diverticulosis of the colon is an out-pouching of colonic mucosa through weakened layers of muscle in the colon wall. The incidence of diverticular increases after the age of 40 [101]. While in itself benign, complications of diverticular disease include diverticulitis, which is the inflammation or infection of diverticula, and painless bleeding, which may be life threatening.

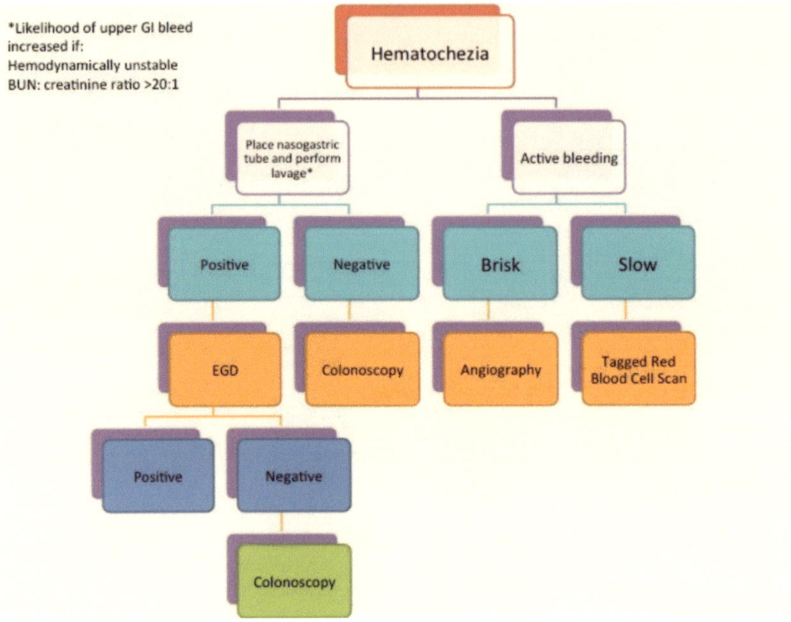

Figure 15. Suggested algorithm by Parekh et al. for the role of colonoscopy in the evaluation of a hemodynamically stable LGIB [100].

Therefore, it is important for the endoscopist to inform the patient of symptoms of potential complications of diverticular disease.

Colonic angioectasias, previously referred to as arteriovenous malformations or angiodysplasias, are a common source of lower gastrointestinal bleeding [102]. They can often times be difficult to identify if not actively bleeding. Figure 16 is an example of colonic diverticula and an angioectasia seen endoscopically.

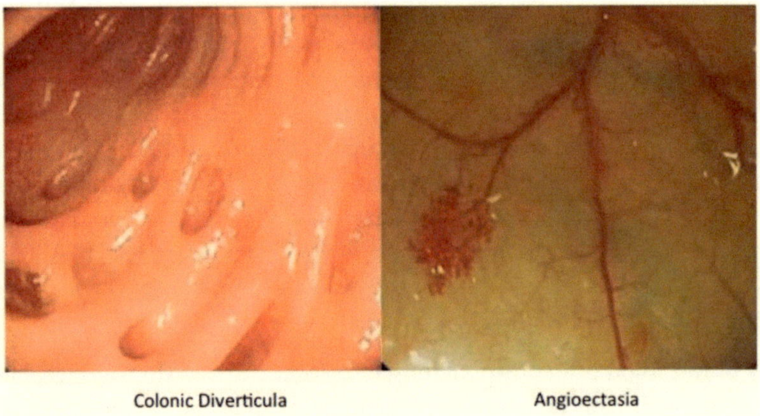

Figure 16. Colonic diverticula and an angioectasia seen endoscopically.

http://dx.doi.org/10.5772/61256

6. Hemorrhoids and anal fissures

Hemorrhoids are vascular structures in the anal canal that act as cushions to help with stool control [103]. When they become swollen or inflamed, internal hemorrhoids (above the dentate line) can present as painless rectal bleeding. External hemorrhoids can result in pain when thrombosed, or painful bleeding if ulceration occurs from pressure necrosis [103]. Skin tags may be evidence of prior thrombosed external hemorrhoids.

An anal fissure is a linear tear or crack in the distal anal canal. It often presents as painful defecation. Initially it usually involves only the epithelium and progresses to include the full thickness of the anal mucosa. Figure 17 is an example of an internal hemorrhoid, external hemorrhoid, skin tag, and an anal fissure.

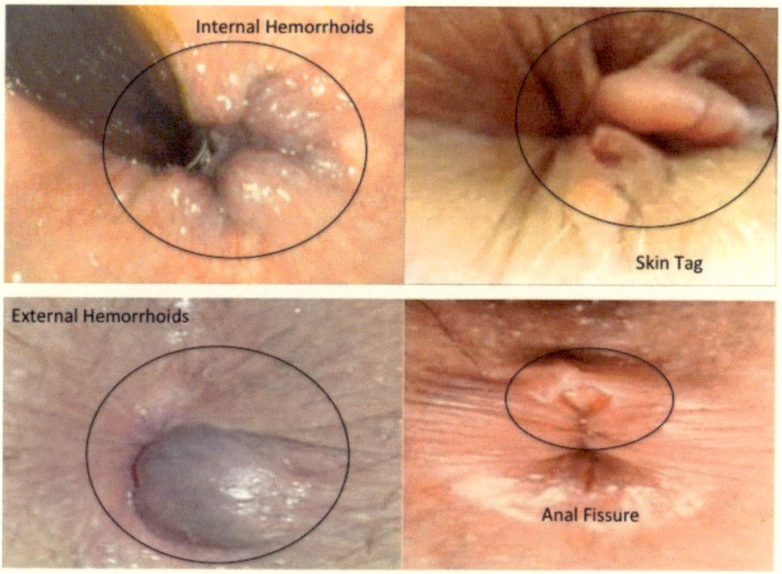

Figure 17. Internal hemorrhoid, external hemorrhoid, skin tag, and an anal fissure.

7. Conclusion

Colonoscopy is important in the diagnosis and therapeutic management of several disease states. To date, colonoscopy remains the gold standard in colorectal cancer prevention. It is the cornerstone in the diagnosis and therapeutic management of IBD, particularly with the recent paradigm shift in the therapeutic management of IBD stressing the importance of endoscopic remission in addition to symptomatic remission. In addition, a thorough colonoscopic exam can aid in the diagnosis of other non-IBD colitides. In the acute setting, findings during colonoscopy are not only crucial in diagnosing the underlying etiology but also driving therapeutic management. As technology evolves and indications for colonoscopy expand, it becomes increasingly more crucial for the clinical endoscopist to be knowledgeable of normal and pathologic findings during colonoscopy.

Author details

Parth J. Parekh and Sanjay K. Sikka*

*Address all correspondence to: ssikka2@tulane.edu

Department of Internal Medicine, Division of Gastroenterology and Hepatology, Tulane University, New Orleans, LA, USA

References

[1] Wolff WI. Colonoscopy: History and development. Am J Gastroenterol. 1989;84(9): 1017-25.

[2] Rex DK, Rahmani EY, Haseman JH, Lemmel GT, Kaster S, Buckley JS. Relative sensitivity of colonoscopy and barium enema for detection of colorectal cancer in clinical practice. Gastroenterology. 1997;112(1):17-23.

[3] Winawer SJ, Zauber AG, Fletcher RH, et al. Guidelines for colonoscopy surveillance after polypectomy: A consensus update by the US Multi-Society Task Force on Colorectal Cancer and the American Cancer Society. CA Cancer J Clin. 2006;56(3):143-59.

[4] Siegel R, Desantis C, Jemal A. Colorectal cancer statistics, 2014. CA Cancer J Clin. 2014;64(2):104-17.

[5] Torre LA, Bray F, Siegel RL, Ferlay J, Lortet-tieulent J, Jemal A. Global cancer statistics, 2012. CA Cancer J Clin. 2015;65(2):87-108.

[6] Winawer SJ, Zauber AG, Ho MN, et al. Prevention of colorectal cancer by colonoscopic polypectomy. The National Polyp Study Workgroup. N Engl J Med. 1993;329(27):1977-81.

[7] Zauber AG, Winawer SJ, O'brien MJ, et al. Colonoscopic polypectomy and long-term prevention of colorectal-cancer deaths. N Engl J Med. 2012;366(8):687-96.

[8] Bressler B, Paszat LF, Chen Z, Rothwell DM, Vinden C, Rabeneck L. Rates of new or missed colorectal cancers after colonoscopy and their risk factors: a population-based analysis. Gastroenterology. 2007;132(1):96-102.

[9] Pickhardt PJ, Nugent PA, Mysliwiec PA, Choi JR, Schindler WR. Location of adenomas missed by optical colonoscopy. Ann Intern Med. 2004;141(5):352-9.

[10] Van gelder RE, Nio CY, Florie J, et al. Computed tomographic colonography compared with colonoscopy in patients at increased risk for colorectal cancer. Gastroenterology. 2004;127(1):41-8.

[11] Lieberman DA, Weiss DG, Harford WV, et al. Five-year colon surveillance after screening colonoscopy. Gastroenterology. 2007;133(4):1077-85.

[12] Martínez ME, Baron JA, Lieberman DA, et al. A pooled analysis of advanced colorectal neoplasia diagnoses after colonoscopic polypectomy. Gastroenterology. 2009;136(3):832-41.

[13] Pancione M, Remo A, Colantuoni V. Genetic and epigenetic events generate multiple pathways in colorectal cancer progression. Patholog Res Int. 2012;2012:509348.

[14] Luo Y, Wong CJ, Kaz AM, et al. Differences in DNA methylation signatures reveal multiple pathways of progression from adenoma to colorectal cancer. Gastroenterology. 2014;147(2):418-29.e8.

[15] The Paris endoscopic classification of superficial neoplastic lesions: esophagus, stomach, and colon: November 30 to December 1, 2002. Gastrointest Endosc. 2003;58(6 Suppl):S3-43.

[16] O'brien MJ, Winawer SJ, Zauber AG, et al. The National Polyp Study. Patient and polyp characteristics associated with high-grade dysplasia in colorectal adenomas. Gastroenterology. 1990;98(2):371-9.

[17] Binmoeller KF, Bohnacker S, Seifert H, Thonke F, Valdeyar H, Soehendra N. Endoscopic snare excision of "giant" colorectal polyps. Gastrointest Endosc. 1996;43(3): 183-8.

[18] Lieberman D, Moravec M, Holub J, Michaels L, Eisen G. Polyp size and advanced histology in patients undergoing colonoscopy screening: Implications for CT colonography. Gastroenterology. 2008;135(4):1100-5.

[19] Van doorn SC, Hazewinkel Y, East JE, et al. Polyp morphology: An interobserver evaluation for the Paris classification among international experts. Am J Gastroenterol. 2015;110(1):180-7.

[20] Leung WK, Lo OS, Liu KS, et al. Detection of colorectal adenoma by narrow band imaging (HQ190) vs. high-definition white light colonoscopy: A randomized controlled trial. Am J Gastroenterol. 2014;109(6):855-63.

[21] Jin XF, Chai TH, Shi JW, Yang XC, Sun QY. Meta-analysis for evaluating the accuracy of endoscopy with narrow band imaging in detecting colorectal adenomas. J Gastroenterol Hepatol. 2012;27(5):882-7.

[22] East JE, Ignjatovic A, Suzuki N, et al. A randomized, controlled trial of narrow-band imaging vs. high-definition white light for adenoma detection in patients at high risk of adenomas. Colorectal Dis. 2012;14(11):e771-8.

[23] Mizuno K, Kudo SE, Ohtsuka K, et al. Narrow-banding images and structures of microvessels of colonic lesions. Dig Dis Sci. 2011;56(6):1811-7.

[24] Winawer SJ, Zauber AG. The advanced adenoma as the primary target of screening. Gastrointest Endosc Clin N Am. 2002;12(1):1-9, v.

[25] Mattar M, Frankel P, David D, et al. Clinicopathologic significance of synchronous and metachronous adenomas in colorectal cancer. Clin Colorectal Cancer. 2005;5(4): 274-8.

[26] Karlitz JJ, Hsieh MC, Liu Y, et al. Population-based lynch syndrome screening by microsatellite instability in patients ≤50: Prevalence, testing determinants, and result availability prior to colon surgery. Am J Gastroenterol. 2015.

[27] Worthley DL, Leggett BA. Colorectal cancer: Molecular features and clinical opportunities. Clin Biochem Rev. 2010;31(2):31-8.

[28] Kakar S, Deng G, Cun L, Sahai V, Kim YS. CpG island methylation is frequently present in tubulovillous and villous adenomas and correlates with size, site, and villous component. Hum Pathol. 2008;39(1):30-6.

[29] Rosty C, Hewett DG, Brown IS, Leggett BA, Whitehall VL. Serrated polyps of the large intestine: current understanding of diagnosis, pathogenesis, and clinical management. J Gastroenterol. 2013;48(3):287-302.

[30] Rex DK, Ahnen DJ, Baron JA, et al. Serrated lesions of the colorectum: Review and recommendations from an expert panel. Am J Gastroenterol. 2012;107(9):1315-29.

[31] Spring KJ, Zhao ZZ, Karamatic R, et al. High prevalence of sessile serrated adenomas with BRAF mutations: A prospective study of patients undergoing colonoscopy. Gastroenterology. 2006;131(5):1400-7.

[32] Sweetser S, Smyrk TC, Sinicrope FA. Serrated colon polyps as precursors to colorectal cancer. Clin Gastroenterol Hepatol. 2013;11(7):760-7.

[33] Anderson JC. Pathogenesis and management of serrated polyps: Current status and future directions. Gut Liver. 2014;8(6):582-9.

[34] Weston AP, Campbell DR. Diminutive colonic polyps: Histopathology, spatial distribution, concomitant significant lesions, and treatment complications. Am J Gastroenterol. 1995;90(1):24-8.

[35] Butterly L, Robinson CM, Anderson JC, et al. Serrated and adenomatous polyp detection increases with longer withdrawal time: Results from the New Hampshire Colonoscopy Registry. Am J Gastroenterol. 2014;109(3):417-26.

[36] Anderson JC, Butterly LF, Goodrich M, Robinson CM, Weiss JE. Differences in detection rates of adenomas and serrated polyps in screening versus surveillance colonoscopies, based on the new hampshire colonoscopy registry. Clin Gastroenterol Hepatol. 2013;11(10):1308-12.

[37] Tadepalli US, Feihel D, Miller KM, et al. A morphologic analysis of sessile serrated polyps observed during routine colonoscopy (with video). Gastrointest Endosc. 2011;74(6):1360-8.

[38] Higuchi T, Sugihara K, Jass JR. Demographic and pathological characteristics of serrated polyps of colorectum. Histopathology. 2005;47(1):32-40.

[39] Provenzale D, Garrett JW, Condon SE, Sandler RS. Risk for colon adenomas in patients with rectosigmoid hyperplastic polyps. Ann Intern Med. 1990;113(10):760-3.

[40] Dave S, Hui S, Kroenke K, Imperiale TF. Is the distal hyperplastic polyp a marker for proximal neoplasia? J Gen Intern Med. 2003;18(2):128-37.

[41] Rex DK, Smith JJ, Ulbright TM, Lehman GA. Distal colonic hyperplastic polyps do not predict proximal adenomas in asymptomatic average-risk subjects. Gastroenterology. 1992;102(1):317-9.

[42] Lin OS, Schembre DB, Mccormick SE, et al. Risk of proximal colorectal neoplasia among asymptomatic patients with distal hyperplastic polyps. Am J Med. 2005;118(10):1113-9.

[43] Weston AP, Campbell DR. Diminutive colonic polyps: Histopathology, spatial distribution, concomitant significant lesions, and treatment complications. Am J Gastroenterol. 1995;90(1):24-8.

[44] Calva D, Howe JR. Hamartomatous polyposis syndromes. Surg Clin North Am. 2008;88(4):779-817, vii.

[45] Choi YS, Suh JP, Lee IT, et al. Regression of giant pseudopolyps in inflammatory bowel disease. J Crohns Colitis. 2012;6(2):240-3.

[46] Maldonado TS, Firoozi B, Stone D, Hiotis K. Colocolonic intussusception of a giant pseudopolyp in a patient with ulcerative colitis: a case report and review of the literature. Inflamm Bowel Dis. 2004;10(1):41-4.

[47] Wyse J, Lamoureux E, Gordon PH, Bitton A. Occult dysplasia in a localized giant pseudopolyp in Crohn's colitis: A case report. Can J Gastroenterol. 2009;23(7):477-8.

[48] Popiolek DA, Kahn E, Procaccino JA, Markowitz J. Nodular neuronal hyperplasia: A distinct morphologic type of pseudopolyp in inflammatory bowel disease. Arch Pathol Lab Med. 1998;122(2):194-6.

[49] Leighton JA, Shen B, Baron TH, et al. ASGE guideline: Endoscopy in the diagnosis and treatment of inflammatory bowel disease. Gastrointest Endosc. 2006;63(4):558-65.

[50] Sulz MC, Bertolini R, Frei R, Semadeni GM, Borovicka J, Meyenberger C. Multipurpose use of the over-the-scope-clip system ("Bear claw") in the gastrointestinal tract: Swiss experience in a tertiary center. World J Gastroenterol. 2014;20(43):16287-92.

[51] Fefferman DS, Farrell RJ. Endoscopy in inflammatory bowel disease: Indications, surveillance, and use in clinical practice. Clin Gastroenterol Hepatol. 2005;3(1):11-24.

[52] Chatzicostas C, Koutroubakis IE, Tzardi M, Roussomoustakaki M, Prassopoulos P, Kouroumalis EA. Colonic tuberculosis mimicking Crohn's disease: Case report. BMC Gastroenterol. 2002;2(1):10.

[53] Lee SK, Kim BK, Kim TI, Kim WH. Differential diagnosis of intestinal Behçet's disease and Crohn's disease by colonoscopic findings. Endoscopy. 2009;41(1):9-16.

[54] Del val JH. Old-age inflammatory bowel disease onset: A different problem? World J Gastroenterol. 2011;17(22):2734-9.

[55] Rameshshanker R, Arebi N. Endoscopy in inflammatory bowel disease when and why. World J Gastrointest Endosc. 2012;4(6):201-11.

[56] Kim B, Barnett JL, Kleer CG, Appelman HD. Endoscopic and histological patchiness in treated ulcerative colitis. Am J Gastroenterol. 1999;94(11):3258-62.

[57] Bernstein CN, Shanahan F, Anton PA, Weinstein WM. Patchiness of mucosal inflammation in treated ulcerative colitis: A prospective study. Gastrointest Endosc. 1995;42(3):232-7.

[58] Jevon GP, Madhur R. Endoscopic and histologic findings in pediatric inflammatory bowel disease. Gastroenterol Hepatol (N Y). 2010;6(3):174-80.

[59] Tontini GE, Vecchi M, Pastorelli L, Neurath MF, Neumann H. Differential diagnosis in inflammatory bowel disease colitis: State of the art and future perspectives. World J Gastroenterol. 2015;21(1):21-46.

[60] Lemmens B, Arijs I, Van assche G, et al. Correlation between the endoscopic and histologic score in assessing the activity of ulcerative colitis. Inflamm Bowel Dis. 2013;19(6):1194-201.

[61] Freeman HJ. Natural history and clinical behavior of Crohn's disease extending beyond two decades. J Clin Gastroenterol. 2003;37(3):216-9.

[62] Nikolaus S, Schreiber S. Diagnostics of inflammatory bowel disease. Gastroenterology. 2007;133(5):1670-89.

[63] Kaiser AM. Discussion of "Backwash ileitis is strongly associated with colorectal carcinoma in ulcerative colitis". Gastroenterology. 2002;122(1):245-6.

[64] Haskell H, Andrews CW, Reddy SI, et al. Pathologic features and clinical significance of "backwash" ileitis in ulcerative colitis. Am J Surg Pathol. 2005;29(11):1472-81.

[65] Daperno M, D'haens G, Van assche G, et al. Development and validation of a new, simplified endoscopic activity score for Crohn's disease: The SES-CD. Gastrointest Endosc. 2004;60(4):505-12.

[66] Ferrante M, Colombel JF, Sandborn WJ, et al. Validation of endoscopic activity scores in patients with Crohn's disease based on a post hoc analysis of data from SONIC. Gastroenterology. 2013;145(5):978-986.e5.

[67] Khanna R, Bouguen G, Feagan BG, et al. A systematic review of measurement of endoscopic disease activity and mucosal healing in Crohn's disease: Recommendations for clinical trial design. Inflamm Bowel Dis. 2014;20(10):1850-61.

[68] Park HS, Han DS, Ro YO, Eun CS, Yoo KS. Does lymphocytic colitis always present with normal endoscopic findings? Gut Liver. 2015;9(2):197-201.

[69] Nomura E, Kagaya H, Uchimi K, et al. Linear mucosal defects: a characteristic endoscopic finding of lansoprazole-associated collagenous colitis. Endoscopy. 2010;42 Suppl 2:E9-10.

[70] Couto G, Bispo M, Barreiro P, Monteiro L, Matos L. Unique endoscopy findings in collagenous colitis. Gastrointest Endosc. 2009;69(6):1186-8.

[71] Sato S, Matsui T, Tsuda S, et al. Endosocopic abnormalities in a Japanese patient with collagenous colitis. J Gastroenterol. 2003;38(8):812-3.

[72] Giardiello FM, Bayless TM, Yardley JH. Collagenous colitis. Compr Ther. 1989;15(2): 49-54.

[73] Pardi DS, Smyrk TC, Tremaine WJ, Sandborn WJ. Microscopic colitis: A review. Am J Gastroenterol. 2002;97(4):794-802.

[74] Alfadda AA, Storr MA, Shaffer EA. Eosinophilic colitis: Epidemiology, clinical features, and current management. Therap Adv Gastroenterol. 2011;4(5):301-9.

[75] Al samman M, Haque S, Long JD. Strongyloidiasis colitis: A case report and review of the literature. J Clin Gastroenterol. 1999;28(1):77-80.

[76] Liu LX, Chi J, Upton MP, Ash LR. Eosinophilic colitis associated with larvae of the pinworm Enterobius vermicularis. Lancet. 1995;346(8972):410-2.

[77] Chandrasekhara V, Arslanlar S, Sreenarasimhaiah J. Whipworm infection resulting in eosinophilic colitis with occult intestinal bleeding. Gastrointest Endosc. 2007;65(4): 709-10.

[78] Friedberg JW, Frankenburg FR, Burk J, Johnson W. Clozapine-caused eosinophilic colitis. Ann Clin Psychiatry. 1995;7(2):97-8.

[79] Anttila VJ, Valtonen M. Carbamazepine-induced eosinophilic colitis. Epilepsia. 1992;33(1):119-21.

[80] Lange P, Oun H, Fuller S, Turney JH. Eosinophilic colitis due to rifampicin. Lancet. 1994;344(8932):1296-7.

[81] Bridges AJ, Marshall JB, Diaz-arias AA. Acute eosinophilic colitis and hypersensitivity reaction associated with naproxen therapy. Am J Med. 1990;89(4):526-7.

[82] Jiménez-sáenz M, González-cámpora R, Linares-santiago E, Herrerías-gutiérrez JM. Bleeding colonic ulcer and eosinophilic colitis: a rare complication of nonsteroidal anti-inflammatory drugs. J Clin Gastroenterol. 2006;40(1):84-5.

[83] Saeed SA, Integlia MJ, Pleskow RG, et al. Tacrolimus-associated eosinophilic gastroenterocolitis in pediatric liver transplant recipients: role of potential food allergies in pathogenesis. Pediatr Transplant. 2006;10(6):730-5.

[84] Martin DM, Goldman JA, Gilliam J, Nasrallah SM. Gold-induced eosinophilic enterocolitis: Response to oral cromolyn sodium. Gastroenterology. 1981;80(6):1567-70.

[85] Clouse RE, Alpers DH, Hockenbery DM, Deschryver-kecskemeti K. Pericrypt eosinophilic enterocolitis and chronic diarrhea. Gastroenterology. 1992;103(1):168-76.

[86] Barbie DA, Mangi AA, Lauwers GY. Eosinophilic gastroenteritis associated with systemic lupus erythematosus. J Clin Gastroenterol. 2004;38(10):883-6.

[87] Ahmad M, Soetikno RM, Ahmed A. The differential diagnosis of eosinophilic esophagitis. J Clin Gastroenterol. 2000;30(3):242-4.

[88] Avgerinos A, Bourikas L, Tzardi M, Koutroubakis IE. Eosinophilic gastroenteritis associated with Churg-Strauss syndrome. Ann Gastroenterol. 2012;25(2):164.

[89] Huguier M, Barrier A, Boelle PY, Houry S, Lacaine F. Ischemic colitis. Am J Surg. 2006;192(5):679-84.

[90] Church J, Kao J. Bedside colonoscopy in intensive care units: indications, techniques, and outcomes. Surg Endosc. 2014;28(9):2679-82.

[91] Zuckerman GR, Prakash C, Merriman RB, Sawhney MS, Deschryver-kecskemeti K, Clouse RE. The colon single-stripe sign and its relationship to ischemic colitis. Am J Gastroenterol. 2003;98(9):2018-22.

[92] Zou X, Cao J, Yao Y, Liu W, Chen L. Endoscopic findings and clinicopathologic characteristics of ischemic colitis: A report of 85 cases. Dig Dis Sci. 2009;54(9):2009-15.

[93] Sultan M, Ramprasad J, Jensen MK, Margolis D, Werlin S. Endoscopic diagnosis of pediatric acute gastrointestinal graft-versus-host disease. J Pediatr Gastroenterol Nutr. 2012;55(4):417-20.

[94] Aslanian H, Chander B, Robert M, et al. Prospective evaluation of acute graft-versus-host disease. Dig Dis Sci. 2012;57(3):720-5.

[95] Crowell KR, Patel RA, Fluchel M, Lowichik A, Bryson S, Pohl JF. Endoscopy in the diagnosis of intestinal graft-versus-host disease: Is lower endoscopy with biopsy as

effective in diagnosis as upper endoscopy combined with lower endoscopy? Pediatr Blood Cancer. 2013;60(11):1798-800.

[96] Xu CF, Zhu LX, Xu XM, Chen WC, Wu DP. Endoscopic diagnosis of gastrointestinal graft-versus-host disease. World J Gastroenterol. 2008;14(14):2262-7.

[97] Strate LL, Ayanian JZ, Kotler G, Syngal S. Risk factors for mortality in lower intestinal bleeding. Clin Gastroenterol Hepatol. 2008;6(9):1004-10.

[98] Chait MM. Lower gastrointestinal bleeding in the elderly. World J Gastrointest Endosc. 2010;2(5):147-54.

[99] Farrell JJ, Friedman LS. Review article: The management of lower gastrointestinal bleeding. Aliment Pharmacol Ther. 2005;21(11):1281-98.

[100] Parekh PJ, Buerlein RC, Shams R, Vingan H, Johnson DA. Evaluation of gastrointestinal bleeding: Update of current radiologic strategies. World J Gastrointest Pharmacol Ther. 2014;5(4):200-8.

[101] Comparato G, Pilotto A, Franzè A, Franceschi M, Di mario F. Diverticular disease in the elderly. Dig Dis. 2007;25(2):151-9.

[102] Management of gastrointestinal angiodysplastic lesions (GIADs): A systematic review and meta-analysis. The American Journal of Gastroenterology. 2014;109(4):474.

[103] Sanchez C, Chinn BT. Hemorrhoids. Clin Colon Rectal Surg. 2011;24(1):5-13.

Section 3

Looking Ahead

Chapter 6

Building up the Future of Colonoscopy – A Synergy between Clinicians and Computer Scientists

Jorge Bernal, F. Javier Sánchez, Cristina Rodríguez de Miguel and Gloria Fernández-Esparrach

Additional information is available at the end of the chapter

http://dx.doi.org/10.5772/61012

Abstract

Recent advances in endoscopic technology have generated an increasing interest in strengthening the collaboration between clinicians and computers scientist to develop intelligent systems that can provide additional information to clinicians in the different stages of an intervention. The objective of this chapter is to identify clinical drawbacks of colonoscopy in order to define potential areas of collaboration. Once areas are defined, we present the challenges that colonoscopy images present in order computational methods to provide with meaningful output, including those related to image formation and acquisition, as they are proven to have an impact in the performance of an intelligent system. Finally, we also propose how to define validation frameworks in order to assess the performance of a given method, making an special emphasis on how databases should be created and annotated and which metrics should be used to evaluate systems correctly.

Keywords: Intelligent systems, Image properties, Validation, Clinical drawbacks, Endoluminal scene description

1. Introduction

1.1. Motivation

During the last few years there has been an increasing effort in exploring the use of intelligent systems to assist and provide additional information to clinicians in the different stages of an intervention. In this context, we can find in the literature systems aiming at assisting the clinician in in-vivo diagnosis such as KARDIO proposed in [1], which can automatically analyze electrocardiograms, or methods that provide with data to help in the detection and diagnosis of breast [2] or prostate cancer [3]. The spread use of Computed Tomography has elicited a new set of methods that help clinicians in intervention planning as exposed in [4]. For instance, we can find systems which allow clinicians to follow the fastest and safest way to target a pulmonary lesion [5], perform laparoscopic surgery [6] or systems such as [7] in the domain of transcatheter aortic valve implantations. However, there is scarce experience with intelligent systems applied to endoscopy where there are only a few methods such as the works presented in [8] in the context of colonoscopy quality assessment which analyzes how clinical procedures have been performed to provide quality scores.

Endoscopic technology has rapidly evolved in the last decade and current equipment allows clinicians to observe the whole endoluminal scene in high definition and, moreover, makes it possible to get different views of the same scene for further analysis by applying automatic techniques of chromoendoscopy [9] as narrow band imaging (NBI) –proposed in [10]-, the Fujinon Intelligent Chromo-Endoscopy (FICE) presented in [11] or Pentax I-scan, which was published in [12]. These advances in endoscopy imaging have generated an increasing interest in strengthening partnerships between clinicians and computer scientists to build applications that can solve some of the challenges that colonoscopy procedures still present nowadays.

It is clear that this potential collaboration between these two domains of knowledge needs from each part to acknowledge the challenges that the analysis of colonoscopy images present related to their area of expertise. Related to this, clinicians need to identify which of the existing drawbacks could be mitigated with the aid of image processing tools and computer scientists must define clearly what can be achieved by means of image processing to provide clinicians with feasible and clinically applicable solutions. Endoscopy imaging analysis present some challenges that are not limited to the ones that the characterization of anatomical structures for detection or diagnosis purposes present; aspects that are rarely covered by existing methods such as image acquisition and formation should be considered as they are proven to have an impact on the output of a given method [13].

Considering this, the focus of this chapter is to present new advances on computer vision methods for colonoscopy and to identify potential clinical issues that may be solved with the aid of computer vision. As it can be observed, this chapter is not written from either a pure clinical or technical point of view but as a way to couple the necessities and challenges of each of the domains in order to build up feasible and clinically applicable systems.

2. Introduction to colonoscopy challenges

2.1. A brief history of endoscopy

The history of endoscopy, as stated in [14], starts in 1805 with P. Bozzini and his attempts to construct a cystoscope (See Table 1). Although this first endoscope was considered as having failed, the principles incorporated in its design - a light source, a reflective surface (lens) and a series of specula (mirrors)- are the basis of current endoscopes. The technical challenges posed since then have been overcome with the collaboration of physicians, engineers, scientists and optical experts among others. The progress has been slow but constant and initially rigid instruments have been changed by flexible endoscopes; candles and lamps have been replaced by electric filaments and, for vision, single lenses have been supplanted by optic fibers.

Year	Authorship	Development
1805	Philipp Bozzini (Physician)	Design of the first endoscope (Lichtleiter). Illumination is provided by candles.
1825	Pierre Solomon Ségalas (Urologist)	Design of an urethro-cystic speculum that incorporates mirrors for projecting light along the tube.
1827	John D. Fisher (Physician)	Development of a cystoscope. His principal innovation is the inclusion of a double convex lens to amplify the image.
1853	Antonin Jean Desormeaux (Urologist)	Demonstration of the first functional endoscope (cystoscope). Candles are replaced by mixture of alcohol and turpentine for illumination.
1865	Francis Richard Cruise (Urologist)	Improvement of the illumination using camphor and petrol and redesigns the lens and lamp system.
1867	Julius Brück (Dentist)	Design of an unusual instrument that uses a lamp lit by electric current.
1868	Adolf Kussmaul (Surgeon)	Attempt at the creation of the first gastroscopy using a rigid instrument based upon sword swallowers.
1870	Gustav Trouvé (Engineer)	Construction of the first electrical endoscopic instrument with optical system: the polyscope (mostly for laryngeal observations).
1877	Max Nitze (Urologist) Fritz Leiter (Manufacturer)	Development the first effective rigid endoscope that incorporates an optical system and an incandescent platinum wire lamp at the end of the cystoscope.
1880	David Newman (Surgeon)	Incorporation of the Edison incandescent lamp into a cystoscope.
1881	Johann Von Mikulicz (Surgeon) Fritz Leiter (Manufacturer)	Development the first practical and functional esophagoscope.
1894	Howard A. Kelly (Gynecologist)	Introduction the first long (30 cm) rigid rectosigmodoscope.
1911	Michael Hoffmann (Physician)	Proposal of a solution to the problem of bending light using multiple prisms and lenses and applies this concept to gastroscopy. This is the first attempt to construct a flexible gastroscope.
1911	Hans Elsner (Physician)	Construction of the first rigid gastroscope.
1922	Rudolf Schindler (Gastroenterologist)	Building of the second rigid gastroscope
1930	Heinrich Lamm (Medical student)	Images are successfully transmitted through glass fibers.

Year	Authorship	Development
1932	Rudolf Schindler (Gastroenterologist) Georg Wolf (Manufacturer)	Development of the first semiflexible gastroscope. Schindler is considered the founder of modern endoscopy.
1940	Cameron Surgical Co.	The first flexible gastroscope is made in the USA: the *Cameron Schindler Endoscope*.
1948	Edward B. Benedict (Surgeon)	Development of the operating gastroscope by incorporating both a biopsy forceps and a suction tube within the gastroscope itself.
1948	Harry Segal (Physician) James Watson (Physician)	Production of a viable endoscopic photographic system.
1952	Tatsuno Uji (Engineer)	Design of a miniature gastrocamera that can be introduced into the stomach.
1957	Basil Hirschowitz (Gastroenterologist) Larry Curtiss (Physicist)	Introduction of the first fiber optic gastroscope.
1960	Machida Endoscope Co. Olympus Optical Co.	Development of the first prototypes of flexible colonoscopes.
1971	William I. Wolff (Surgeon) Hiromi Shinya (Surgeon)	Performance of the first polypectomy with a wire loop snare.
1975	Masahiro Tada (Gastroenterologist)	Description of the first magnifying colonoscope.
1983	Welch Allyn Inc.	Development of an electronic sensor or charge coupled device that is inserted at the tip of the endoscope.
2002	Olympus Co.	HD endoscopes

Table 1. Evolution of endoscopy as a result of collaboration of different disciplines

Shortly after having successfully traversed the esophagus and reached the stomach, the assessment of the duodenum, small intestine and colon were the next steps that were progressively addressed and achieved. Other needs were also identified and solved: first, the evolution from diagnostic to operating endoscopes that allowed obtaining biopsies; second, the need of preserving the image of the lesion which was observed. The latter not only reflected clinical needs but also documentation and educational requirements. At that point, several corporations became involved in the development of endoscopic instrumentation and they also designed cameras specifically for endoscopic usage.

Once the fiber optic endoscope was established as a reality by late 1960s, numerous design modifications were performed with the collaboration of physicians in order to augment the utility of the device and increase its resolution. The decade of 1970 witnessed a series of rapid technological advances where a number of instrumental manufactures including ACMI, Olympus Optical Company and Machida Endoscope Company included a variety of innovations (length, flexibility, channel size...) that improved the performance of the instrument. In 1983 video endoscopy was introduced as the logical consequence of technical advances in microelectronics and all current endoscopes are based on this technology. Video endoscopy allows an easy exploration, instant image acquisition and further storage confirming its utility not only for clinical practice but also for educational purposes.

2.2. High definition endoscopy (The quality of image matters)

In the last years, most of the developments in endoscopy have been focused on improving the quality of images, as it is the case of high definition (HD) endoscopes that use a 1080-line television and a high resolution charge coupled device with up to 1.3 million pixels. This allows the acquisition and storage of images with double the resolution of normal television. Other capabilities available in some endoscopes are the following:

- Wide angle: the endoscope has a field of vision of 170º (30% more than the conventional model) that is supposed to improve the detection of lesions hidden behind the folds;
- Electronic zoom: that achieves a ×80–100 maximum effect;
- Narrow band imaging (NBI): a modification in the light beam enhances visualization of the network of the mucosa providing contrast and acting as a substitute of chromoendoscopy. This system offers the possibility to switch from conventional white light to blue NBI light alternatively (see Fig.1).

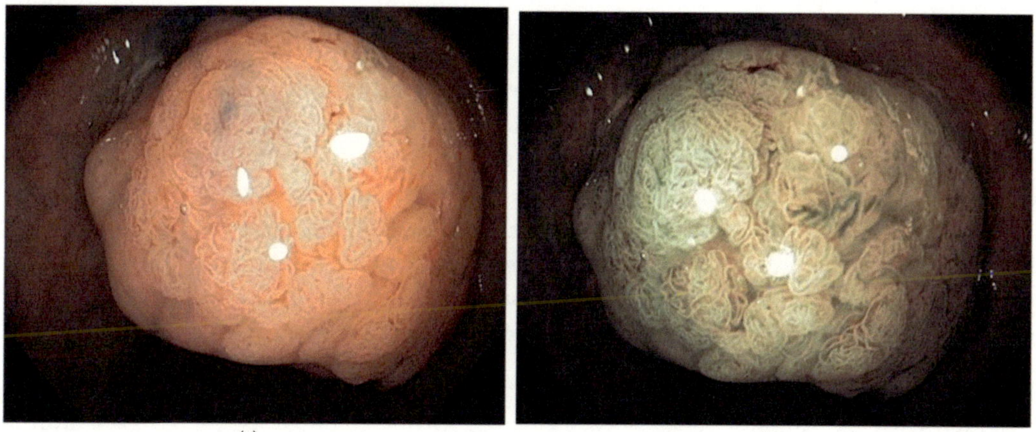

(a) (b)

Figure 1. Example of a same polyp observed with white light (a) and NBI (b).

HD endoscopes (particularly those with magnification function) facilitate the demonstration of the mucosal architectural and vascular patterns that are altered in dysplastic lesions as it can be observed in Fig.2. With regards to the detection rate of lesions, although it is logical to assume that a higher resolution endoscope could provide better results, the results of several studies [15, 16] do not support this hypothesis.

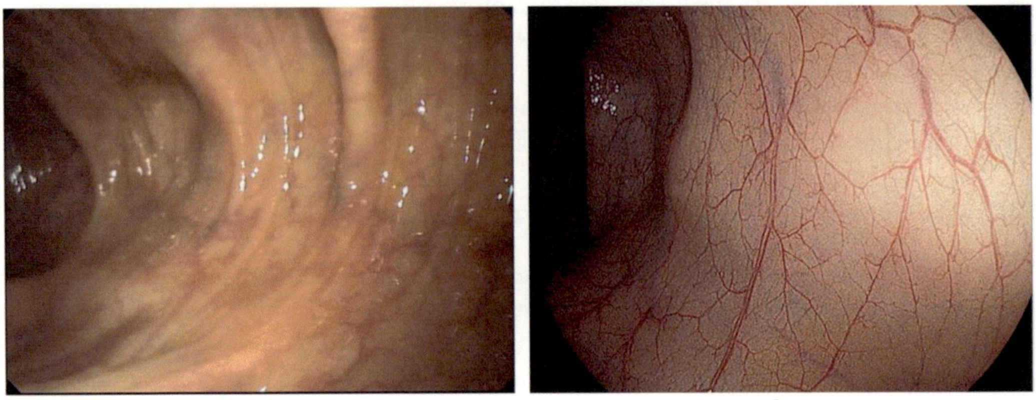

(a) (b)

Figure 2. Example of a colonoscopy frame observed with conventional endoscope (a) and with high definition endoscope (b).

2.3. The problem of colonic polyps

Colorectal cancer (CRC) is a serious health problem in the general population and it is considered that at least two thirds of CRC develop through the adenoma–carcinoma pathway. Consequently, screening with colonoscopy for CRC and its precursor lesion has become an increasingly practice, as shown in [17]. Several actions have been proposed to optimize colonoscopy such as ensuring colon perfect preparation and carrying out a thorough examination of the mucosa which would imply a longer withdrawal inspection time, as indicated in [18].

However, colonoscopy still presents some drawbacks being the most relevant the polyp miss-rate -reported to be as high as 22%- resulting in a lack of total effectiveness [19]. The rate of polyps missed increases significantly in smaller sized polyps (2% for adenomas ≥ 10 mm versus 26% for adenomas < 5 mm) and this has a clinical impact, not only because the prevalence of high-grade dysplasia increases with the size as exposed in [20] but because of the risk of having an interval cancer. Interval colorectal cancers are described as cancers occurring after a negative screening test or examination and they are an important indicator of the quality and effectiveness of CRC screening and surveillance, as stated in [21].

The diagnosis of dysplasia has practical consequences on the management of polyps. There is general consensus on removing all polyps detected during colonoscopy but size is a limiting factor for endoscopic polypectomy. Therefore, having a histological diagnostic of presumption is very useful in order to make the decision of performing or not a polypectomy. In this regard, there are several classifications (NICE, Kudo...) that predict the histology of the lesion based on the characteristics of the image. Kudo [22] proposes a gross classification of pit patterns into 7 types: type I and II pit patterns are characteristic of non-neoplastic lesions such as normal mucosa or hyperplastic polyps whereas pattern types IIIS, IIIL, IV, and a subset of VI are intramucosal neoplastic lesions such as adenoma or intramucosal carcinoma and lesions with a type VN pattern and a subset of type VI suggest deep invasive carcinoma (see Fig. 3).

http://dx.doi.org/10.5772/61012

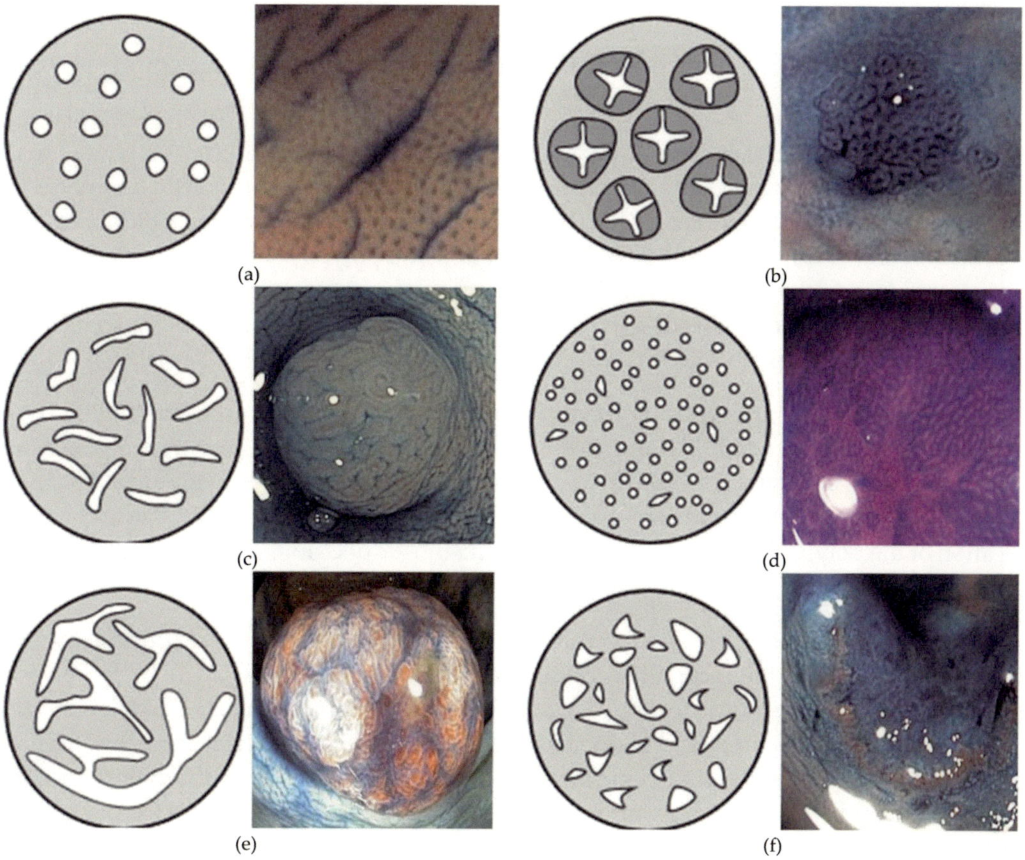

Figure 3. Examples of Kudo neoplastic lesion classification: (a) Type I; (b) Type II; (c) Type IIIL; (d) Type IIIS; (e) Type IV and (f) Type V.

As this classification applies for magnification endoscopy, when it is used with conventional endoscopy the results are worse. Contrarily, NICE is an international classification of colorectal tumors on the basis of NBI observation either with or without use of a magnifying endoscope [23]. NICE is a simple categorical classification defining three different types based on three characteristics: (i) lesion color; (ii) micro vascular architecture; and (iii) surface pattern. Type 1 is considered an index for hyperplastic lesions, type 2 an index for adenoma or mucosal/ submucosal scanty invasive carcinoma, and type 3 an index for deeply submucosal-invasive carcinoma The problem with these classifications is that diagnostic derives from a subjective visual analysis and requires specific training and a high degree of experience.

Finally, the precise location of the polyps is another meaningful drawback of colonoscopy, not only when planning a surgery but also during successive colonoscopies. This limitation is especially remarkable in the presence of several polyps. In this case, an exhaustive analysis of the surface and boundaries of the polyp could be very helpful.

2.4. Identification of potential collaborative research areas between clinicians and computer scientists

Considering the mentioned drawbacks of colonoscopy, three potential areas in which computer science may play a role have been identified:

- Automatic polyp detection and localization: one of the exposed drawbacks is related to the difficulty on detecting certain types of polyps such as small or flat lesions. Flat polyps can be detected with the support of CT [24, 25] although its detection supposes additional patient radiation and is limited by the size. Detection of small polyps cannot be undertaken with the help of CT as the current available resolution makes it impossible to detect polyps with size smaller than 10 mm as stated in [26], therefore the diagnosis in these cases should only rely on endoscopic exploration.

- Polyp classification: the decision of performing polypectomy is commonly taken by an estimation of the size and histology of the detected lesion. This estimation is commonly made by means of visual observation and therefore incorporates some degree of subjectivity. In this context, a system that can objectively provide an estimation of the size and classification of the polyp could allow taking in-vivo diagnostic decisions and this would optimize the treatment timing.

- Patients lesion follow-up and endoscopy navigation: there is a necessity expressed by some clinicians regarding the recognition of the area that a lesion occupies, which can be useful for two different reasons: 1) for the case of polyps that have not been removed, an univocal recognition of the lesion would allow the study of the evolution of the lesion; 2) an accurate recognition of the marks that clinicians leave to identify the area of the polyp once it is removed would allow the exploration of areas nearby the lesion to search for new pathologies.

3. Image processing challenges for the analysis of colonoscopy videos

In order to provide clinicians with meaningful applications, the content of colonoscopy videos and frames must be thoroughly analyzed by computer scientists to search for lesions or indicators defined by clinicians. In this context, the majority of the literature has been focused on developing methods to characterize accurately the different elements of the endoluminal scene, paying special attention to polyps. Although it is clear that anatomical landmarks recognition is essential for application development, the acquisition and generation of high quality images is also crucial for computer vision methods in order to work as they are intended. For instance, the presence of image artifacts has been proven to have an impact in the performance of polyp localization methods, as shown in [13].

Considering this we present in this section a summary of the most important challenges that a given computer vision method must face in order to provide with efficient support to clinicians. We have divided the challenges in two groups: those related to image acquisition

http://dx.doi.org/10.5772/61012

and formation and those related to the characterization of anatomical structures needed to build up the clinicians' support system.

3.1. Identification of endoscopy image particularities with impact in image processing analysis

Videos that endoscopes generate are created following common television standards in a way such they can provide with sufficiently moving image quality while allowing for efficient resource management in case endoscopy images and videos are stored for later inspection. It is important to mention that quality in this case is understood under human's observer point of view but not under computer visions; for instance there are some image processing techniques automatically performed – i.e. sharpening - that may improve how images are observed but, as they modify the original image, they create new elements that affect an automatic analysis by means of computer vision methods. Some of the features that can affect the performance of a computer vision method are listed below and in table 2:

- *Illumination effects:* The way colonoscope illuminates the scene produces an axial illumination which tends to generate *specular highlights* on shiny surfaces such as the mucosa. Mucosa is covered by a thin watery film which generates many specular highlights when it is illuminated in a perpendicular direction to its surface. Specular highlights position will vary with little movements of the colonoscope which will change the angle at which mucosa is illuminated therefore areas of the mucosa affected by specularities will change rapidly. The presence of specular highlights difficult strongly image processing [13] as they appear as very prominent structures which also hinder color and texture information about the surfaces in which they appear. Moreover, axial illumination introduces also an additional side-effect regarding its *lack of uniformity* in the way structures are illuminated: structures closer to the endoscope will appear brighter than others far from the endoscope (see Fig. 4).

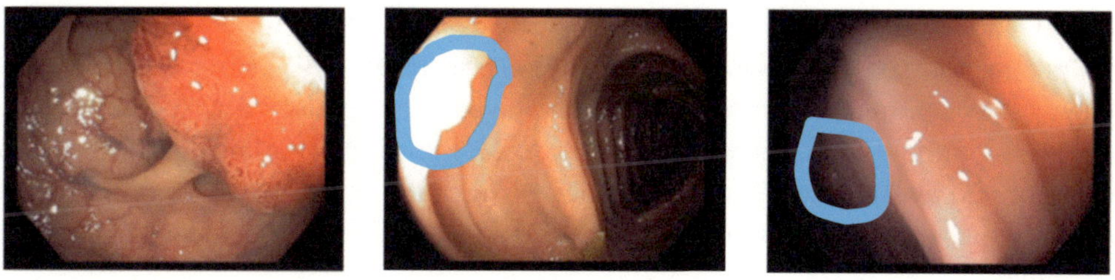

(a) (b) (c)

Figure 4. Examples of illumination effects: (a) specular highlights (b) overexposed polyp and (c) underexposed polyp. Polyps in images b and c are delimited with a blue mask to ease visualization.

- *Sensor acquisition effects: Color phantoms* appear due to temporal misalignment of color channels related to some endoscopes that still use monochrome sensors. In this case, color information is generated by illuminating the scene with the three primary colors (red, green and blue) successively. Consequently, three different images are needed to generate a color image. This process introduces some undesired side-effects associated to camera movement: as we acquire the images in different time instants, specular highlights generated by the light source in each of the three moments will be located in slightly different positions, causing instability in the final color image –Fig. 5(a).

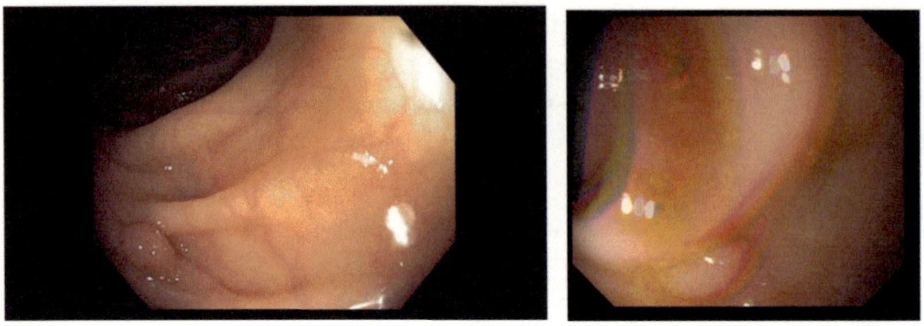

(a) (b)

Figure 5. Effect of channel misalignment due to monochrome sensors: instability in specular highlights position (a) and apparition of color phantoms (b).

Moreover, as each color channel is acquired in different times, the three components (red, green and blue) will not be exactly aligned if the endoscope moves when the image is acquired. This lack of color channel alignment generates artificial color bands in the contours of the structures –Fig. 5(b) - that appear in the image which limits the performance of any color information-based structure characterization method.

- *Image resolution:* Commercial endoscopes generate videos in formats following television standards (PAL for Europe, NTSC for America and Japan). These formats are meant to generate motion images with enough quality to be observed by the general public but also minimizing the size of the information to be transmitted. By acting this way, videos generated by commercial endoscopes can be played in any standard system (TV, personal computers) without needing format conversion. Moreover, the minimization of the amount of transmitted information allows a reduction of the storage needs which is crucial in clinical settings where the amount of resources dedicated to information storage must be efficiently distributed.

Although the use of standard formats presents clear advantages for visualization and storage purposes, it does not benefit image processing by means of computer vision. Video standards offer images with lower resolution than the one that can be achieved by means of commercial cameras. For instance, NTSC standard provides as output 0.3 Megapixels images, HD standard offers images up to 2 Megapixels and a commercial camera easily exceeds 10 Megapixels [27]. Low resolution images lead to a loss of texture information associated to anatomical structures in the endoluminal scene, which can have an impact on the output of structure classification methods -Fig. 6-.

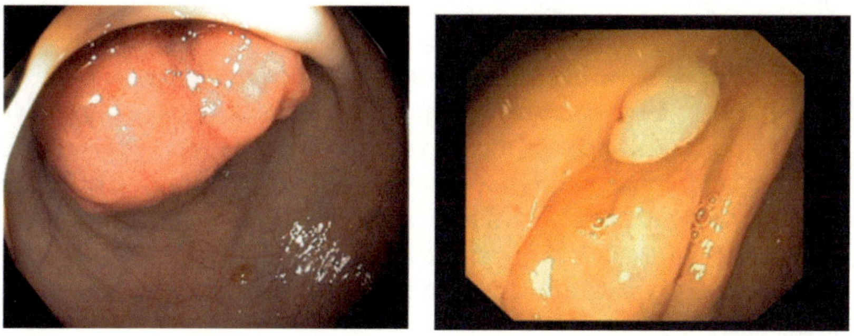

(a) (b)

Figure 6. Different colonoscopy images acquired at different resolutions: (a) high resolution image and (b) low resolution image. We can observe greater texture details in the polyp from the highest resolution image.

- *Image interlacing:* As it has been mentioned before, from all available video standards those with lowest bandwidth –amount of information that needs to be transmitted-requirements are chosen for use in endoscopy. This reduction in bandwidth is achieved by interlacing image lines, which is performed by acquiring odd and even image lines in different time instants. By this we can double the image refresh rate without increasing the size of the information. This also makes video movement appear smoother and more continuous to the human eye but it has a counterpart that affects posterior image processing. The final image provided by the processor will be a mixture of two different images captured in different time instants: even lines will be from the first capture whereas odd lines will come from the second. As with color channel misalignment, interlacing impact will depend on the amount of endoscope movement between the two acquisitions. For instance, if camera moves horizontally we can observe sawtooth profiles in vertical contours, apart from change of position of specular highlights. We show in Fig. 7 a clear example on how interlacing can affect the quality of the image to be processed by, for instance, the apparition of double and shadowy contours surrounding the elements of the image.

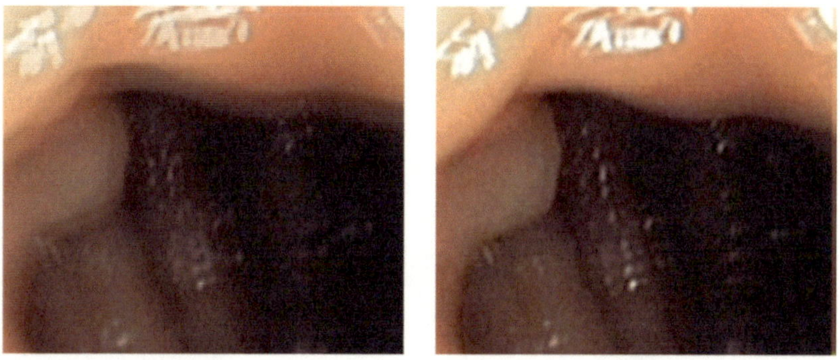

(a) (b)

Figure 7. Impact of interlacing in image quality: (a) Interlaced image and (b) Separate field of an interlaced image.

- *Sharpening:* Endoscopes and video processors include functionalities that improve the quality of the image to be visualized by human observers, aiming to simplify the observation of particular structures in the images. One of the most common techniques is sharpening, which describes a subjective perception of sharpness related to edge contrast in an image. By applying this technique, contours that separate different objects in the image can be more clearly identified and consequently structures can be easily separated –Fig. 8 (b)-. This visualization enhancement [28] comes at a cost in terms of image processing as contour enhancement implies a modification of the original image which increases image noise. Sharpening also generate halos around structures that appear in the image such as specular highlights, as observed in Fig. 8 (b).

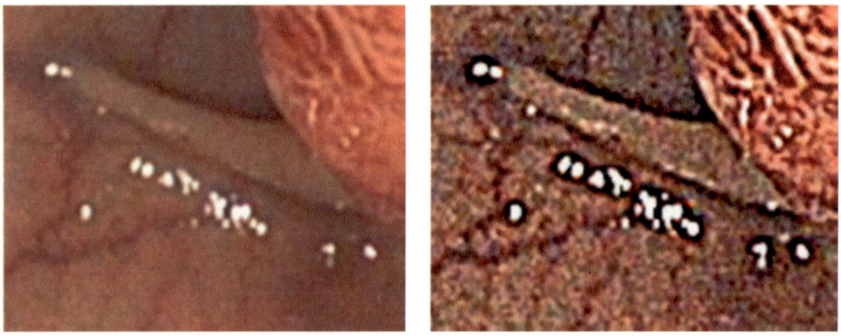

(a) (b)

Figure 8. Examples of sharpening applied on colonoscopy images: (a) Original image and (b) image with sharpening applied.

- *Information overlay:* Video processors associated to endoscope do not present a specific output dedicated to its connection to a personal computer. Considering this, the image that the clinician is observing will be the same that will be stored for later processing. It is common that some information regarding the procedure such as patient information or procedure date is superimposed to the image provided by the colonoscope, as it can be observed in Fig. 9. The presence of this information precludes its use for research purposes, as this data should be anonymzed. Moreover the presence of this information superimposed to the original image may difficult the observation and characterization of structures in the images apart from introducing additional noise and elements (letters, numbers) to the image.

- *Black mask:* Endoscopes automatically add an octagonal or circular black mask surrounding the image acquired by the sensor. This mask covers those regions of the image that are strongly affected by geometric distortions introduced by wide angle optic used in endoscopes. These distortions, similar to fisheye effects present in some cameras, makes structures below the mask appear different to what they are in reality and consequently they should not be analyzed by clinicians. Unfortunately the presence of this black mask affects the performance of image processing methods, as the mask creates strong contours in the separation between the mask and the endoluminal scene, as it can be observed in Fig. 10.

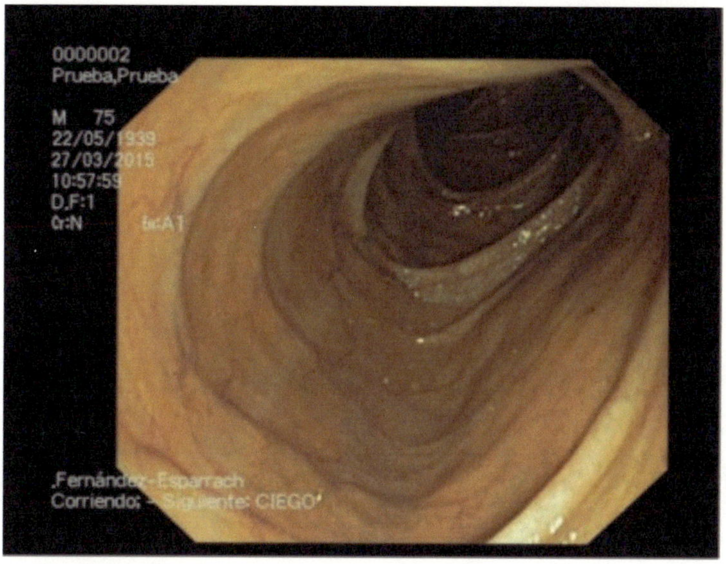

Figure 9. Examples of information overlay in colonoscopy images.

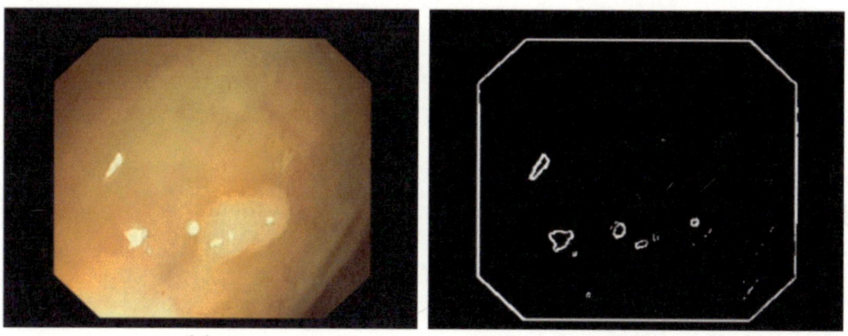

(a) (b)

Figure 10. Impact of black mask in image processing algorithms. (a) shows the original image whereas (b) shows the output of an edge detection algorithm. Note that mask contours appear as strong as structural elements.

- *Data compression:* Image and video data are commonly compressed in order to save storage space but commonly used formats such as MPEG and JPEG lead to information loss along with the introduction of some artifacts they may difficult fine detail processing in images. In this case the lower the compression, the least impact it will have in further image processing.

3.2. Endoluminal scene description challenges

In order to provide with systems that can help clinicians to overcome some of the clinical challenges identified earlier, a description of the elements of the endoluminal scene is needed. We show in Fig.11 an example on how endoluminal scene looks like.

We can make a division of the elements that appear on a given scene into pure anatomical structures (polyps, luminal region, folds, blood vessels or intestinal content) and structures appearing as result of image acquisition and formation processes (specular highlights and black mask). It is clear that a potential intelligent system should focus on the characterization of anatomical structures in order to be clinically useful –being polyps the usual target structure- but, as recent studies demonstrate [29], the consideration of all the elements of the endoluminal scene may result in an improvement of the performance of a given system. Endoluminal structure characterization is not a straightforward task due to three main reasons:

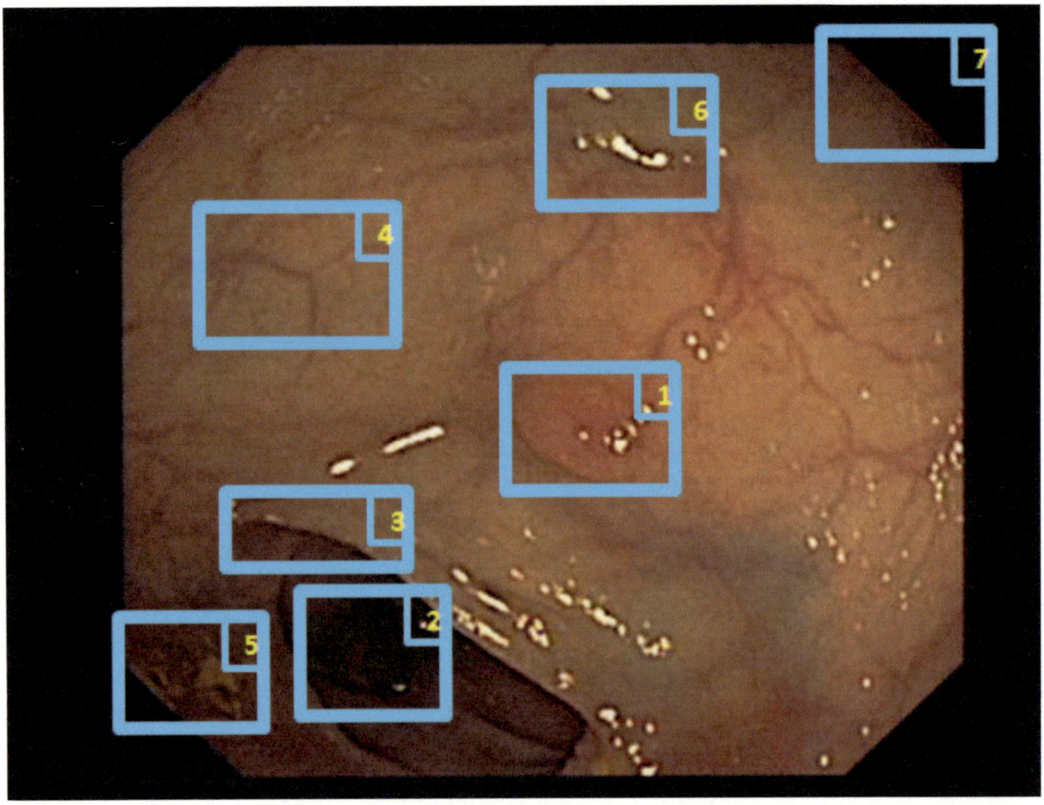

Figure 11. Elements of the endoluminal scene: (1) Polyp; (2) Luminal region; (3) Folds; (4) Blood vessels; (5) Intestinal content; (6) Specular highlights and (7) Black mask.

- *Lack of uniform structure appearance:* Anatomical structures appearance differs greatly in different interventions, which may difficult the development of characterization methods that can be widely applicable. For instance, polyp characterization is challenging because there is not an uniform and unique polyp appearance; in fact, polyp appearance depends greatly on the point of view in which it is observed and we can observe different particularities whether we are observing polyps in zenithal or lateral views –see Fig. 12-.

http://dx.doi.org/10.5772/61012

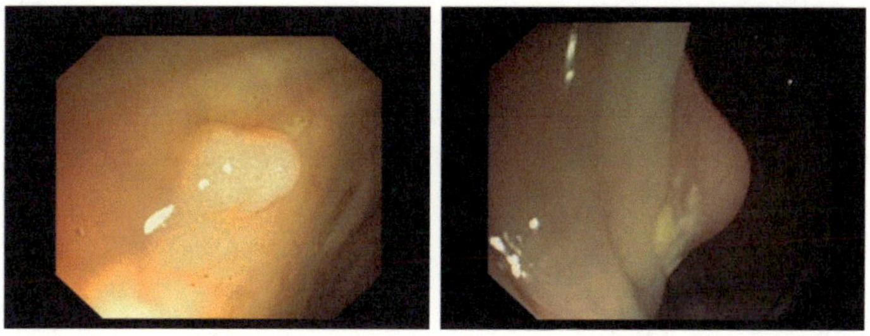

(a) (b)

Figure 12. Variability in polyp appearance: (1) Zenithal view and (2) Lateral view.

Consequently a definition of a model of appearance for a given structure should consider this great variability in order to be widely applicable and, therefore, search for general features that can be attainable for the majority of the cases.

- *Impact of other elements of the scene on a particular element characterization:* Following with the polyp example, the majority of available works rely on polyp characterization from the identification of polyp boundaries but, in terms of image processing, there is not a big difference in terms of contour appearance between polyps, blood vessels and folds, as the three of them provide with similar response to contour detection operators, as it can be observed in Fig. 13. Considering this, a given intelligent system must consider the impact of all present structures when providing a characterization of a particular one and it will need to find additional cues to differentiate between these structures.

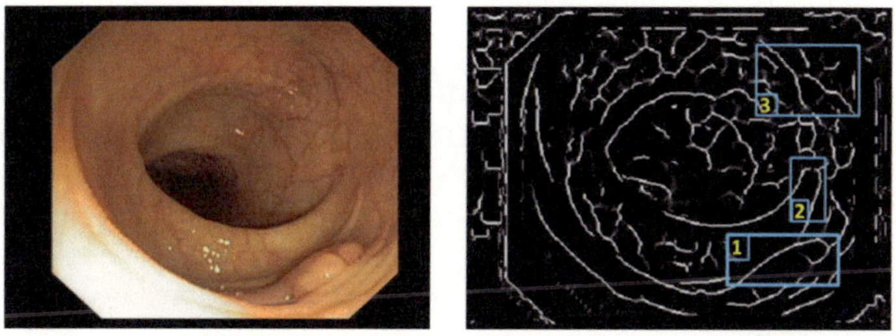

(a) (b)

Figure 13. Example of similarity of response of different structures to a given operator. Number 1 represents a polyp, number 2 a fold and 3 represents blood vessels.

- *Difficulties on the definition of the structural element:* Another challenge is related to the visual definition of the structure itself, that is, sometimes the definition of the element itself is not clear, which makes it difficult to delimit the structure. For instance, recent studies show a great variability between observers when defining the luminal region –demonstrated in [30], which may have an impact on ground truth creation for assessing the performance of a given intelligent system. This difficult on the definition on the structure can also be applied for other elements such as fecal or intestinal content.

4. Equipment setting to favor optimal image processing analysis

We present in this section the optimal settings of clinical equipment to ensure the best possible quality of the images which will be analyzed by the intelligent system.

4.1. Endoscopic equipment settings

Chronologically, the first element to be considered is the configuration of both endoscope and video processor in order to obtain the best possible images for further analysis. In this case we propose the following configuration:

- Disable sharpening options, so we can avoid the apparition of artificial information (halos) surrounding image structure contours along with reducing image noise.
- Disable the superimposition of overlay information such as patient or procedure data to obtain a clean view of the endoluminal scene. This also allows a complete anonymization of the information easing its use for research purposes.
- If possible, allow the endoluminal view to occupy the largest portion of the scene without applying any kind of digital zooming operation.
- Configure storage options to obtain data with the minimum possible compression.

4.2. Image storage and anonymization

We have to consider that image or/and video data will be used in research projects from which several research publications will be generated. Access to this image or video data should be granted to other researchers in order to allow an easier comparison of the performance of different methods. Considering this, no information that can allow an identification of either the patient or the clinician should be provided in neither the images or in the metadata associated to them –such as time and date of image capture or endoscopy used-, preventing the association of a given image to a patient, clinician or hospital.

Considering the amount of endoscopic interventions performed in a hospital in a year, images or videos that are stored tend to be compressed. This compression has already been mentioned to have implications for image processing methods so; if possible, the configuration with less possible compression should be chosen.

4.3. Endoscopic naviagation guidelines

Endoscope movement when images are acquired impacts the quality of the images that are obtained. If there is no scope movement, effects such as interlacing or color phantoms can be almost inexistent -Fig. 14 (a)-. Considering this, we propose still images acquisition to be made being both the scope and the elements of the endoluminal scene static. For the case of video acquisition we suggest slow and smooth endoscope progression through the patient in order to maximize the reduction of movement-related artifacts generation.

http://dx.doi.org/10.5772/61012

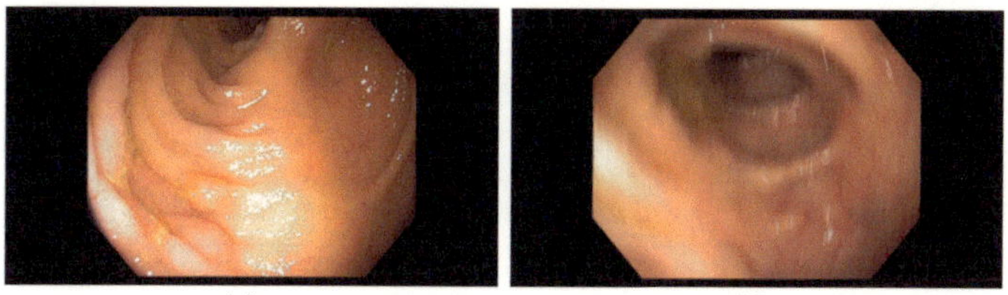

(a) (b)

Figure 14. Difference in image quality related to endoscope movement when acquiring images: (a) still endoscope vs. (b) moving endoscope.

It is clear that even by considering all the suggestions expressed, there will still be a minor movement of the scope between the two time instants in which odd and even lines of the final image are acquired. In order to mitigate the impact of interlacing and to avoid loss of image resolution we propose to make a real-time analysis of the images when they are acquired in order to store only the one which less interlacing impact. This analysis will be made by comparing consecutive frames, where the difference in content between them is so minimal that there is no point on storing them all, considering the small changes that will appear in images extracted from a 30 frames per second video. In case interlacing can still be perceived, its impact can be completely removed by working with one of the two channels of the image [29], although this implies a decrease in final image resolution.

To close this section, we show in Table 2 a summary of the challenges related to image formation and acquisition depicted in Section 3 and our proposal on how to solve/mitigate them. As it can be seen from the table, there are some challenges that cannot be solved by applying specific settings to the devices involved. For instance, those related to image formation are highly device-dependent. In this sense, newer equipment has dedicated sensors for each color channel avoiding the apparition of color phantoms. There are other challenges that must be solved by means of image processing techniques, such as specular highlights. In this sense, the most accepted solution [29] consists of a specular highlight detection followed by a substitution of the pixels in the image belonging to specular highlights by a combination of valid values of neighbor pixels, as it can be observed in Fig. 15. The same operation is applied to mitigate the impact of strong contours created by the black mask.

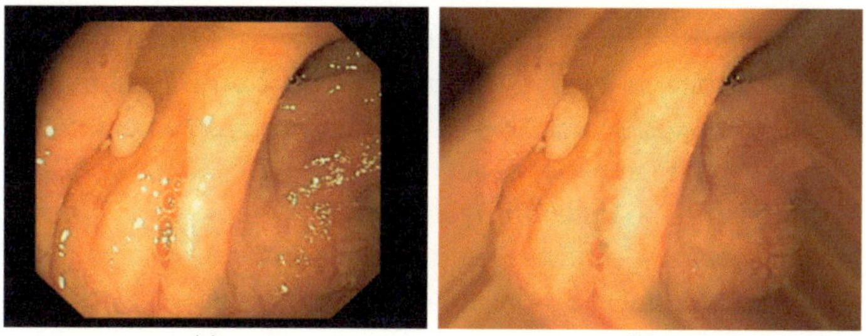

(a) (b)

Figure 15. Application of image processing methods to mitigate impact of specular highlights and black mask. (a) Original image and (b) Processed image.

Source	Challenge		Proposed solution
Image formation	Illumination	Specular highlights	Specular highlights correction
		Lack of uniform illumination	Device-dependent
	Sensor acquisition	Color phantoms	Device-dependent
Image acquisition and visualization	Image acquisition and storage	Image resolution	Stabilization of endoscope, interlacing suppression and use of HD endoscopes
		Image interlacing	Interlacing suppression, neighbor frame frames, endoscope stabilization
	Image visualization capabilities enhancement	Sharpening	Disable sharpening
		Presence of patient and procedure information	Disable overlays
		Black mask	Black mask substitution
		Data compression	Use of lossless compression standards.

Table 2. Summary of image acquisition and formation challenges along with proposal of solutions

5. Current endoluminal scene description methods

We present in this section a review on the most recent works published on the topic of anatomical endoluminal scene elements description.

5.1. Polyps

As they are the main focus of colonoscopy explorations, the majority of already existing intelligent systems for colonoscopy deals with polyp characterization. We divide existing systems according to the application they are built for:

- *Polyp detection:* This group of methods aim to decide whether there is a polyp or not in the image. The majority of the works on polyp detection are built on the principle of applying a given feature detector/descriptor to the image in order to guide detection methods. In this sense, we can divide existing approaches in two groups: (a) shape and (b) texture and color-based. The first group aims to detect polyps by observing specific cues on the contours of the polyp –examples of this can be found in works presented in [31-33], or by fitting candidate objects in the image to the most common shapes that polyps present [34]. Regarding the second group, the use of several general descriptors has been proposed, such as wavelets in [35], local binary patterns in [36] or co-ocurrence matrices [37]. A method combining MPEG-7 texture and color descriptors was proposed in [38]. One big drawback of descriptor-based methods is that they tend to need of an exhaustive training and they are

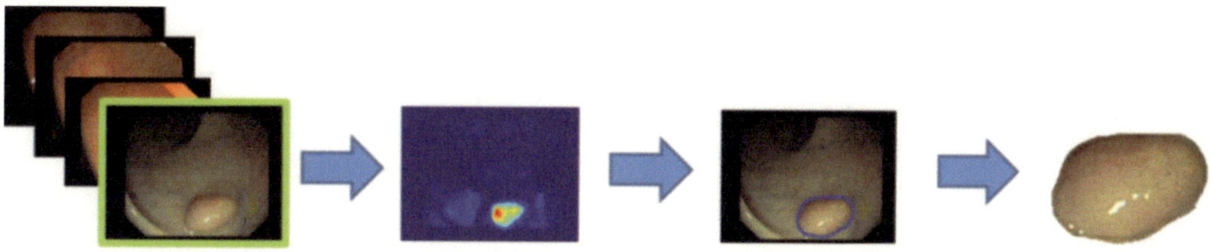

Figure 16. Example of the output of each polyp characterization group of algorithms.

very sensitive to parameter tuning. Finally the work published in [39] combines shape and texture features to build up a polyp detection method which also considers spatial and temporal adjacency information present in colonoscopy videos.

- *Polyp localization/highlighting:* These methods are focused on highlighting the area of the image more likely to contain a polyp. Considering this, they can be understood as a subgroup of polyp detection method but, in this case, with the objective to establish the area of the image where the polyp is. These methods rely on the definition of a model of polyp appearance and on the exploration of low-level features of the image –in this case, the definition of polyp boundaries in terms of valley information- in order to provide with methods that can be applied in the intervention rooms. Some examples of these methods can be found in the works of Bernal et al [13, 29].

- *Polyp segmentation:* In this case the objective is to delimit the region of the image that the polyp occupies. The majority of available works deal with polyp segmentation in CT images -such as the works depicted in [40,41] -, which can also be useful to provide further features of the polyp such as its size, although considering CT limitations regarding small polyps visibility as mentioned in Section2. Recent works on white light colonoscopy exploit the output from polyp localization methods in order to delimit the final polyp region [42], providing accurate results that could be directly applicable in the intervention room without additional radiation of the patient. Finally there are some recent works [43] that deal with polyp segmentation using narrow-band imaging; preliminary results are promising although its usefulness is restricted to the availability of this imaging modality.

- *Polyp characterization/classification*: The aim of these methodologies concerns lesion characterization according to the content of the polyp region. In this case the objective is to aid clinicians in in-vivo diagnosis and some of the existing works aim to provide automatic lesion labeling using previously-mentioned classifications such as NICE [23] or KUDO [22]. These systems would benefit from an accurate localization and segmentation of the polyp region in order to find features that best discriminate between different polyp types.

As it can be seen from the classification exposed above, a potential intelligent system with applicability in the intervention room could easily use a system from each of the four groups in order to build up a computer-aided diagnosis tool. We show in Fig. 16 a graphical example of such a system. In a first stage the system will automatically decide which frames contain a polyp and which region of the frame contains the polyp. From this, an accurate segmentation of the polyp region will be obtained in order to extract meaningful features to help in the classification process.

5.2. Luminal area

Luminal area is defined as the interior space of a tubular structure, such as the intestine. The detection of the lumen and its position can be crucial in both intervention and post-intervention time.

On the one hand, an accurate detection of the lumen region during in-vivo intervention may be useful to discard areas of the image with low visibility –Fig. 17(a) - in order to save computation time for other interesting regions of the image as proposed in [44]. Lumen detection can also be helpful to guide the clinician inside the intestine by pointing out which direction he/she should take to progress. On the other hand, lumen characterization in post-intervention can be used to discard frames for further revision: frames where the proportion of lumen out of the entire image is large can be related to the progression of the colonoscope through the gut but, conversely, frames where the amount of lumen presence is low may potentially indicate areas of the image where the physician has paid more attention. This can be useful to obtain summary videos of the whole procedure. Lumen characterization has been an active topic of research in several endoscopy image modalities such as optical –works of [45] and [46] - and virtual colonoscopy [47]. The main reasoning behind the majority of the luminal region characterization methods is the assumption that lumen is the darkest region of the image and from this seed region growing algorithms are built in order to find lumen boundaries.

5.3. Blood vessels

Blood vessels are the part of the circulatory system that transports blood through the body and they can be identified by their tree-like shape with ramifications. The characterization of these branching structures has been reported in domains such as retinal image analysis [48] or palm prints recognition [49]. Blood vessels characterization in colonoscopy images can be useful in two domains: helping in polyp localization and segmentation tasks, as it has been proven in [13, 29, 42], and as key points to be used in potential follow-up methods, as proposed in [50]. Regarding the former, a mitigation of blood vessels related valleys by using contrast properties of blood vessels contours has been proven to be useful to improve polyp localization segmentation, as in some images -Fig. 17(b)- blood vessels can be identified easier than polyp boundaries. Concerning the latter, we could think of a univocal characterization of blood vessels branching patterns using methods such as the one proposed in [51] to recognize a same region during different interventions.

5.3.1. Folds

Haustral folds represent folds of mucosa within the colon. They are formed by circumferential contraction of the inner muscular layer of the colon. In the context of intelligent systems for colonoscopy, folds characterization can play a key role in polyp characterization tasks. In this sense, we have to consider that the fold contours appearance in colonoscopy images is very similar to the one of polyps. We can observe in Fig. 17 (c) that folds and polyp contours present similar appearance but different levels of curvature; consequently, an accurate identification of folds could lead to an improvement in polyp characterization tasks. Some recent works build up advances model of polyp appearance to discriminate polyp contours from folds by considering desirable properties of polyp contours such as concavity, completeness or continuity, as proposed in [13].

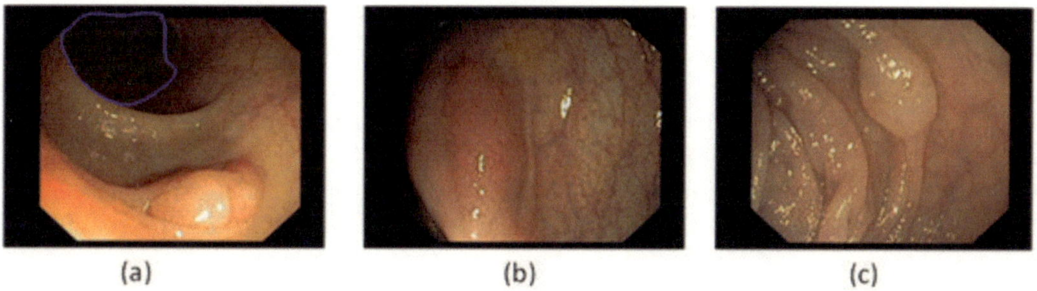

Figure 17. Effect of endoluminal scene structures in polyp characterization: (a) Luminal region (delimited by a blue mask); (b) Blood vessels and (c) Folds.

5.4. Fecal content

Apart from the elements that have already been covered, there are more elements that can appear in the endoluminal scene as a result of bad patient preparation. In this sense high presence of intestinal content is considered by clinicians as an indicator to decide whether a procedure has to be repeated or not as no clinician or computer vision method would work with very low quality images. Moreover, there are some cases when the presence of fecal content can affect the output of computer vision methods, as it was shown in [13]. Therefore an accurate identification of fecal content in colonoscopy images could be used to provide automatic indicators of the quality of patients' preparation.

6. Building up validation frameworks for intelligent systems

One of the main problems when assessing the performance of the different available intelligent systems for colonoscopy is that the majority of them are tested on private databases, which makes it difficult to observe the differences in performance between them and to extrapolate its functioning in other environments. Moreover, it is very difficult to compare performance levels of different methods as each of them proposes or uses different evaluation metrics which, for some cases, can be only used with a specific application in mind. Considering this two problems, we present in this section our proposal for a complete validation framework covering from database and ground truth creation to the definition of the metrics to be used to evaluate a given method.

6.1. Database creation

In order to validate and assess the performance of a computer vision method, this has to be tested in a set of images covering as many possible cases of study. For instance, if we want our method to be able to characterize polyps from all the types present in Paris classification our database should contain several examples from each of the classes that are defined there. Apart from the original images, a ground truth should also be provided. This ground truth will be used to assess the performance of the method and its configuration will depend on the concrete experiment. Following the same example used before, for polyp localization purposes the ground truth should consist of a binary image where pixels in white should correspond to those pixels which are part of the polyp. If the output of a given method falls in the white pixels of the image, the method will be performing as expected. As it can be seen there are two processes involved when creating databases for intelligent systems validation: the selection of the cases to be included in the database and the creation of the corresponding ground truth.

Regarding the selection of the cases, in order the use of a method can be extended outside research domain, these cases should represent the clinical variability that the clinician can find during interventions. In case we have several types of elements to be characterized, the database should contain as many different examples as possible for all the possible classes. It is important to mention than the more different the examples, the more robust will be our method and the better it will perform once a new case of study is to be analyzed. By doing this if we achieve that a given method offers good performance in our database it will be easy to extrapolate its performance in a potential clinical application.

There is one branch of computer vision known as machine learning which involves method training in a set of images and a posterior testing of this method in a different set of images, once its performance has been optimized in the training stage. Considering this, the size of the database should permit the division in training and testing examples and we should define our database in a way such representative examples of all the possible cases are present both in training and testing databases. The final size of the database should allow extracting statistically significant conclusions. In clinical trials, a variability of less of 10 % is not considered as relevant as stated in [52], being variability calculated as the inverse of the square root of the number of samples –N- in our database. Considering this, the minimum size of the database should be of 100 images.

Once database has been defined, ground truth must be created to validate the performance of the methods. The definition of this ground truth is clearly application dependent: for instance if we are developing a polyp detection method the ground truth may only consist of an excel file indicating for each frame whether there is a polyp or not in the image but for a polyp segmentation method we would need a binary image representing the structure to be segmented, as it can be seen in Fig. 18.

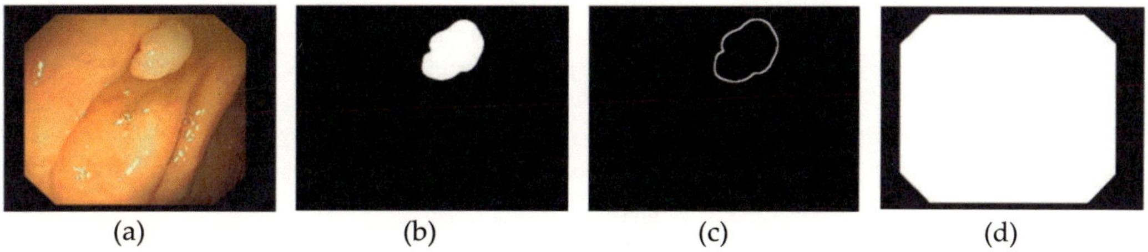

Figure 18. Possible contents of a polyp segmentation database: (a) Original image; (b) Polyp mask; (c) Polyp contour mask and (d) Black mask.

Image-based ground truth are commonly created using image editing software such as Microsoft Paint or Adobe Photoshop, although there is an increasing use of specific tools such as ImageJ [53] which allows the creation of segmentation ground truths by marking a few points in the image. Concerning ground truth creation, it should be created either by clinicians or by experts under clinicians' supervision. Having more than one ground truth per image is recommendable for validation purposes as a way to avoid possible subjectivity in ground truth creation. This allows performing statistical tests and also to assess whether the performance of a given method is within inter-observer variability. If clinical conclusions are meant to be extracted from the performance of intelligent systems, clinical metadata should be provided. For instance, if we want to assess the performance of a polyp classification method, apart from the mask representing where the polyp in the image is, clinicians should provide which is the class of the polyp (i.e., KUDO type I).

Currently there are only, up to our knowledge, three different databases related to colonoscopy image analysis: two of them consisting of still images showing a polyp - CVC-ColonDB and CVC-ClinicDB- and another - ASU-Mayo Clinic polyp database-, which consists of full colonoscopy videos with and without polyps. The first two databases are meant for the validation of model of appearance for polyps to ease polyp localization and segmentation whereas the latter has been developed for the validation of polyp detection algorithms. Currently only CVC-ClinicDB incorporates clinical metadata associated to each polyp, including information regarding polyp size, Paris classification and histological type of polyp. This allows break down of the results according clinical criteria, as exposed in [13]. We introduce the main features of each of the three databases in Table 3.

6.2. Performance metrics

The way a given intelligent system method is validated will depend greatly on what this intelligent system is for. The potential application the system is designed for will define both how database and ground truth need to be generated and the metrics used to assess the performance of the method. In this subsection we propose validation protocols for each of the four main types of intelligent systems reported in the literature.

Database	Number of frames/videos	Ground truth content
CVC-ColonDB	380 frames from 15 different sequences with a polyp	For each image with a polyp the following images are provided: 1) original image; 2) polyp mask; 3) non-informative regions mask and 4) polyp contour.
CVC-ClinicDB	612 frames from 29 different sequences with a polyp.	For each image both the original frame along with a mask covering the polyp are provided. For each polyp, clinical metadata associated is provided (size, Paris classification, histological type of polyp after biopsy) [13]
ASU-Mayo Clinic polyp database	Training set: 20 videos (10 with a polyp and 10 without polyps). Testing set: 18 videos	For each frame of the video a binary image is provided. Absence of polyp in the image can be identified by having a completely black associated image. In case of polyp presence, an approximation of polyp region is provided.

Table 3. Summary of available databases for colonoscopy image analysis

- *Polyp Detection:* A given polyp detection method should provide an output whenever a polyp is present in the image and should not provide any output if there is no polyp.

Performance metrics:

Considering this we propose the use of four different concepts (True Positive (TP), False Positive (FP), True Negative (TN) and False Negative (FN)) which are commonly used in object detection and characterization problems. We present these concepts in Table 4.

Concept	Method	Ground truth
TP	Provides an output	There is a polyp in the image
FP	Provides an output	There is no polyp in the image
TN	Does not provide an output	There is no polyp in the image
FN	Does not provide an output	There is a polyp in the image

Table 4. Explanation of polyp detection metrics

Consequently a good polyp detection method should provide with a high number of TP and TN along the lowest possible number of FN and FP. In order to allow a more clear representation of these results, four different metrics are calculated from TP, FP, TN and FN values:

- Precision, calculated as: $Prec = \frac{TP}{TP + FP}$. It represents the fraction of relevant retrieved information. Regarding polyp detection, it represents the percentage of correct alarms (frames where the method provides an output and the image has a polyp). A low precision rate will be interpreted as the system providing a high number of false alarms.

http://dx.doi.org/10.5772/61012

- Recall, calculated as: $Rec = \frac{TP}{TP + FN}$. Recall represents the fraction of elements to be retrieved that have been successfully retrieved. In our context, represents the fraction of polyps out of the total that have been correctly detected. Considering this, the highest recall the best the detection method.

- Accuracy, calculated as: $Acc = \frac{TP + TN}{TP + FP + TN + FN}$. This measure represents the amount of information that has been correctly labeled. It is useful in cases where positive and negative examples are balanced which is not always the case for polyp detection.

- Specificity, calculated as: $Spec = \frac{TN}{FP + TN}$. This represents how good a polyp detection method is when detecting the absence of polyps. A high number of false alarms can be interpreted as the method being less specific regarding polyp presence.

Finally, a polyp detection method will be considered as clinically useful if it can helps the clinician to detect the polyp. Considering this and assuming that a given sequence contains a polyp, the following metrics can be defined:

- Reaction time: difference in number of frames between first apparition of the polyp in the sequence and the first frame in which a given method provides detection.
- Dwell time: number of frames with a polyp in which the detection method provides detection.

Considering this two metrics, a comparison can be made between the performance of a given automatic method and clinicians, as it was presented in [13]. This can allow the assessment of the potential of a given method to be included to support clinicians in polyp detection tasks.

Ground truth:

Ground truth for polyp detection methods validation can consist in either a text file stating which frames contain a polyp or in a binary mask corresponding to each original frame. In this case the binary mask should represent polyp presence and absence (for instance, an all-black image can represent polyp absence).

- *Polyp localization:* Polyp localization methods aim to extend the information provided by polyp detection methods by not only indicating whether there is a polyp in the image or not, but also indicating where the polyp is within the image.

Performance metrics:

Considering the purpose of localization methods, we cannot use all the four concepts explained before as the use of TN does not make sense in this type of problems as there is always a polyp in the image. In this case several authors [13] propose a more direct performance referred as localization accuracy. Considering that a polyp localization method always provide a potential polyp location, we can define a good localization (GL) whenever the output of the localization method coincides with a polyp. Conversely we define false localization (FL) in the opposite case when the localization proposed by the method falls outside the polyp. Taking this into account, we define localization accuracy as:

$$LAcc = \frac{GL}{GL + FL}$$

In cases where the output of a localization image does not consists of points representing polyp locations but of energy images representing areas with more likelihood of containing a polyp –as it can be seen in Fig. 16- the use of energy concentration metrics seems useful to represent the performance of a method [13]. Considering these two metrics, LAcc and concentration, a good localization method should provide a low number of FL while concentrating the majority of the polyp presence likelihood image inside the polyp mask.

Ground truth:

Ground truth for polyp localization should consist of binary masks representing the area of the image that is occupied by the polyp, as it is shown in Figure 18.

- *Polyp segmentation:* An accurate segmentation of the region that contains the polyp can be useful for both lesion recognition tasks as well as for delimiting the area of the image to be used for lesion classification purposes.

Performance metrics:

We propose the use of common segmentation metrics such as Precision and Recall, as they were defined for polyp detection. In this case we classify each pixel as TP, FP, TN and FN considering methods' output and the ground truth (i.e. a false positive pixel is defined as a pixel in which our method states it is part of the polyp when it is not). In this context, a good polyp segmentation method should provide higher Precision and Recall results (Fig. 19 (b)); a method providing high Precision with low Recall will provide regions that cannot be used for further polyp characterization as they contain lots of non-polyp information (Fig. 19 (c)). Conversely a method providing with high Recall but low Precision values will be useful for polyp description but will leave a lot of useful polyp content out of posterior analysis (Fig. 19 (d)).

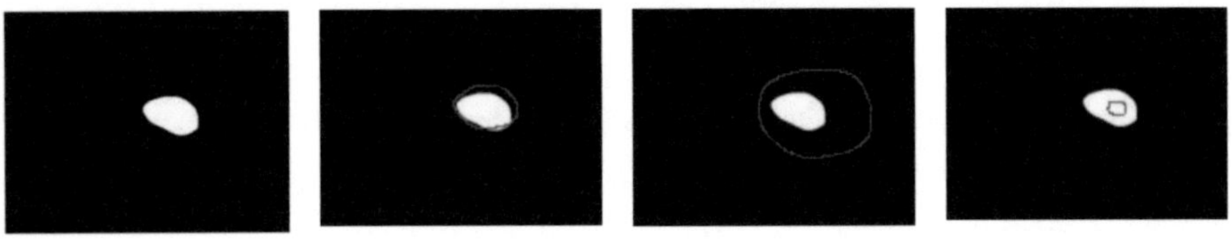

(a) (b) (c) (d)

Figure 19. Interpretation of segmentations: (a) Original ground truth. Segmentation results with (a) good Precision and Recall values; (c) good Precision but low Recall value and (d) low Precision but good Recall value. Mask representing the output of a given method is represented in blue.

Ground truth:

As for the case of polyp localization, ground truth for polyp segmentation should consists of binary masks representing either the area of the image that is occupied by the polyp -Figure 18 (b)- or the contour of the polyp region -Figure 18 (c)-.

http://dx.doi.org/10.5772/61012

- *Polyp classification:* A good polyp classification method should be able to assign the polyp present in the image the same label/class that is attached to the polyp in the ground truth.

Performance metrics:

In this case we can have two different types of evaluation, depending on the number of possible classes that we define: if a polyp can only have two different classes we could evaluate our method by checking whether the output of a method coincides or not with the ground truth; in this case for each image we will have a correct (OK) or incorrect classification (NOK). The accuracy of the system will be calculated as

$$Acc = \frac{OK}{OK + NOK}$$

The second type of evaluation is related to multiclass classification; in this case we can also include studies regarding which classes are more easily identified and which classes are mostly confused over each other. In this last case we can use confusion matrices, similar to the ones presented in [54] to represent the output of a given classification method.

Ground truth:

Ground truth for polyp classification should consist of a label associated to each frame with a polyp; this label must include the given polyp in any of the possible classes defined in the problem.

7. Conclusions

Collaboration between clinicians and computer scientists is crucial for the development of intelligent systems for colonoscopy. Those systems need to be designed to solve real clinical problems if they want to be deployed in clinical environments. Considering this, apart from application development and validation, efforts must be focused on the definition of the aim of the proposed intelligent system.

We have presented in this chapter some of the problems that colonoscopy still present nowadays, being polyp miss-rate the most important of them. Additionally there is a need expressed by clinicians of systems that can allow them to have a first approach to polyp histology, which could be useful to take in-vivo decisions. Considering this we define three possible domains of application of a given intelligent system: polyp detection and localization, polyp classification and development of navigation-assisting and patient follow-up methods.

Once the clinical need is defined, computer scientists must deal with image processing in order to provide with meaningful results. In this context, we have subdivided this problem in two:

image preparation for optimal image processing and endoluminal scene description for intelligent system applications.

Regarding image preparation, one of the main objectives of this chapter was to rise up some concerns about image quality for later processing and clinicians and computer scientists must reach an agreement to obtain images that are useful for both domains. Endoluminal scene description has been proven as a challenging task due to the great variability in structures' appearance throughout different interventions. The majority of bibliographical sources are devoted to polyp characterization, although we have observed an increasing interest in the definition of other elements of the scene, as they have been proven to have an impact in polyp characterization tasks. At this point it is important to mention that there are some aspects that we have not covered in full such as patient preparation although it has a direct consequence on the output of a given intelligent system. In this case we opt to follow the same criteria that clinicians do: if patient preparation is bad neither computer vision nor clinicians would be able to distinguish anything.

The objective of the development of an intelligent system is to take profit of the synergies between clinicians and computer scientists. During the development of a given system, clinicians must provide with data in order to test different methods. We propose in this chapter a validation framework which covers topics such as database and ground truth creation as well as the definition of performance metrics. The proposal of a validation framework including database creation and management along with the definition of standard evaluation metrics can pave the way for a standardized comparison of the performance of intelligent systems which would allow in the future clinicians choose the one that fulfills better their necessities.

The main conclusion that can be extracted from this chapter is that there is indeed room and necessity for the collaboration between these two domains of research. Acknowledging the necessities of each other is meant to play a key role in the development of applicable and deployable intelligent systems for colonoscopy.

Author details

Jorge Bernal[1*], F. Javier Sánchez[1], Cristina Rodríguez de Miguel[2] and Gloria Fernández-Esparrach[2]

*Address all correspondence to: jbernal@cvc.uab.es

1 Computer Science Department at Universitat Autònoma de Barcelona and Computer Vision Center, Barcelona, Spain

2 Endoscopy Unit, Gastroenterology Department, Hospital Clínic, IDIBAPS, CIBEREHD, University of Barcelona, Barcelona, Spain

References

[1] Bratko, I., Mozetič, I., & Lavrač, N. (1990). KARDIO: a study in deep and qualitative knowledge for expert systems. MIT Press. DOI:10.1016/0933-3657(91)90006-W

[2] Wilschut, J. A., Steyerberg, E. W., van Leerdam, M. E., Lansdorp-Vogelaar, I., Habbema, J. D. F., & van Ballegooijen, M. (2011). How much colonoscopy screening should be recommended to individuals with various degrees of family history of colorectal cancer?. Cancer, 117(18), 4166-4174. DOI: 10.1002/cncr.26009

[3] Viswanath, S., Palumbo, D., Chappelow, J., Patel, P., Bloch, B. N., Rofsky, N et al. (2011, March). Empirical evaluation of bias field correction algorithms for computer-aided detection of prostate cancer on T2w MRI. In SPIE Medical Imaging (pp. 79630V-79630V). International Society for Optics and Photonics. DOI:10.1117/12.878813

[4] Bale, R., & Widmann, G. (2007). Navigated CT-guided interventions. Minimally Invasive Therapy & Allied Technologies, 16(4), 196-204. DOI:10.1080/13645700701520578

[5] Schwarz, Y., Greif, J., Becker, H. D., Ernst, A., & Mehta, A. (2006). Real-time electromagnetic navigation bronchoscopy to peripheral lung lesions using overlaid CT images: the first human study. CHEST Journal, 129(4), 988-994. DOI:10.1378/chest.129.4.988

[6] Fernández-Esparrach, G., Estépar, R. S. J., Guarner-Argente, C., Martínez-Pallí, G., Navarro, R., de Miguel, C. R et al. (2010). The role of a computed tomography-based image registered navigation system for natural orifice transluminal endoscopic surgery: a comparative study in a porcine model. Endoscopy, 42(12), 1096. DOI: 10.1055/s-0030-1255824

[7] Grbic, S., Ionasec, R., Mansi, T., Georgescu, B., Vega-Higuera, F., Navab, N., & Comaniciu, D. (2013, April). Advanced intervention planning for Transcatheter Aortic Valve Implantations (TAVI) from CT using volumetric models. In Biomedical Imaging (ISBI), 2013 IEEE 10th International Symposium on (pp. 1424-1427). IEEE. DOI: 10.1109/ISBI.2013.6556801

[8] Thomas-Gibson, S., Bassett, P., Suzuki, N., Brown, G. J., Williams, C. B., & Saunders, B. P. (2007). Intensive training over 5 days improves colonoscopy skills long-term. Endoscopy, 39(9), 818-824. DOI: 10.1055/s-2007-966763

[9] Kiesslich, R., Fritsch, J., Holtmann, M., Koehler, H. H., Stolte, M., Kanzler, S. et al. (2003). Methylene blue-aided chromoendoscopy for the detection of intraepithelial neoplasia and colon cancer in ulcerative colitis. Gastroenterology, 124(4), 880-888. DOI:10.1053/gast.2003.50146

[10] Machida, H., Sano, Y., Hamamoto, Y., Muto, M., Kozu, T., Tajiri, H., & Yoshida, S. (2004). Narrow-band imaging in the diagnosis of colorectal mucosal lesions: a pilot study. Endoscopy, 36(12), 1094-1098. DOI:10.1055/s-2004-826040

[11] Yoshida, Y., Matsuda, K., Sumiyama, K., Kawahara, Y., Yoshizawa, K., Ishiguro, H., & Tajiri, H. (2013). A randomized crossover open trial of the adenoma miss rate for narrow band imaging (NBI) versus flexible spectral imaging color enhancement

(FICE). International journal of colorectal disease, 28(11), 1511-1516. DOI:10.1007/s00384-013-1735-4

[12] Hoffman, A., Kagel, C., Goetz, M., Tresch, A., Mudter, J., Biesterfeld, S. et al. (2010). Recognition and characterization of small colonic neoplasia with high-definition colonoscopy using i-Scan is as precise as chromoendoscopy. Digestive and Liver Disease, 42(1), 45-50. DOI :10.1016/j.dld.2009.04.005

[13] Bernal, J., Śanchez, F. J., Fernández-Esparrach, G., Gil, D., Rodńguez, C., & Vilarin̄o, F. (2015). WM-DOVA Maps for Accurate Polyp Highlighting in Colonoscopy: Validation vs. Saliency Maps from Physicians. Computerized Medical Imaging and Graphics, 43,pp. 99-111. DOI :10.1016/j.compmedimag.2015.02.007

[14] Modlin, I. M. (2000). A brief history of endoscopy. MultiMed.

[15] Pellise, M., Fernández-Esparrach, G., Cardenas, A., Sendino, O., Ricart, E., Vaquero et al. (2008). Clinical impact of wide-angle, high-resolution endoscopy in the diagnosis of colorectal neoplasia in a non-selected population: a prospective randomized controlled trial. Gastrointestinal Endoscopy, 67(5), AB101. DOI :10.1016/j.gie.2008.03.119

[16] Rex, D. K., & Helbig, C. C. (2007). High yields of small and flat adenomas with high-definition colonoscopes using either white light or narrow band imaging. Gastroenterology, 133(1), pp. 42-47. DOI :10.1053/j.gastro.2007.04.029

[17] Quintero, E., Castells, A., Bujanda, L., Cubiella, J., Salas, D., Lanas, Á. et al. (2012). Colonoscopy versus fecal immunochemical testing in colorectal-cancer screening. New England Journal of Medicine, 366(8), pp. 697-706. DOI: 10.1056/NEJMoa1108895

[18] Barclay, R. L., Vicari, J. J., Doughty, A. S., Johanson, J. F., & Greenlaw, R. L. (2006). Colonoscopic withdrawal times and adenoma detection during screening colonoscopy. New England Journal of Medicine, 355(24), pp. 2533-2541. DOI: 10.1056/NEJMoa055498

[19] van Rijn, J. C., Reitsma, J. B., Stoker, J., Bossuyt, P. M., van Deventer, S. J., & Dekker, E. (2006). Polyp miss rate determined by tandem colonoscopy: a systematic review. The American journal of gastroenterology, 101(2), pp. 343-350. DOI:10.1111/j.1572-0241.2006.00390.x

[20] Bretagne, J. F., Manfredi, S., Piette, C., Hamonic, S., Durand, G., & Riou, F. (2010). Yield of high-grade dysplasia based on polyp size detected at colonoscopy: a series of 2295 examinations following a positive fecal occult blood test in a population-based study. Diseases of the Colon & Rectum, 53(3), pp. 339-345. DOI: 10.1007/DCR.0b013e3181c37f9c

[21] Samadder, N. J., Curtin, K., Tuohy, T. M., Pappas, L., Boucher, K., Provenzale, D. et al. (2014). Characteristics of missed or interval colorectal cancer and patient survival:

a population-based study. Gastroenterology, 146(4), pp. 950-960. DOI:10.1053/j.gastro.2014.01.013

[22] Kudo, S. E., Wakamura, K., Ikehara, N., Mori, Y., Inoue, H., & Hamatani, S. (2011). Diagnosis of colorectal lesions with a novel endocytoscopic classification–a pilot study. Endoscopy, 43(10), 869. DOI: 10.1055/s-0030-1256663

[23] Hayashi, N., Tanaka, S., Hewett, D. G., Kaltenbach, T. R., Sano, Y., Ponchon, T. et al. (2013). Endoscopic prediction of deep submucosal invasive carcinoma: validation of the narrow-band imaging international colorectal endoscopic (NICE) classification. Gastrointestinal endoscopy, 78(4), pp. 625-632. DOI:10.1016/j.gie.2013.04.185

[24] Fidler, J. L., Johnson, C. D., MacCarty, R. L., Welch, T. J., Hara, A. K., & Harmsen, W. S. (2002). Detection of flat lesions in the colon with CT colonography. Abdominal imaging, 27(3),pp. 292-300. DOI: 10.1007/s00261-001-0171-z

[25] Fidler, J., & Johnson, C. (2009). Flat polyps of the colon: accuracy of detection by CT colonography and histologic significance. Abdominal imaging, 34(2), pp. 157-171. DOI: 10.1007/s00261-008-9388-4

[26] Johnson, C. D., Chen, M. H., Toledano, A. Y., Heiken, J. P., Dachman, A., Kuo, M. D et al. (2008). Accuracy of CT colonography for detection of large adenomas and cancers. New England Journal of Medicine,359(12), pp. 1207-1217. DOI: 10.1056/NEJMx080041

[27] Poynton, C. (2012). Digital video and HD: Algorithms and Interfaces. Elsevier.

[28] Cambridge in Color: A Learning Community for Photographers. Sharpening: Unsharp Mask. http://www.cambridgeincolour.com/tutorials/unsharp-mask.htm. Last visit: 29/03/2015.

[29] Bernal, J., Sánchez, F. J., & Vilariño, F. (2013, July). Impact of image preprocessing methods on polyp localization in colonoscopy frames. In Engineering in Medicine and Biology Society (EMBC), 2013 35th Annual International Conference of the IEEE (pp. 7350-7354). IEEE. DOI:10.1109/EMBC.2013.6611256

[30] Sánchez, C., Bernal, J., Sánchez, F.J., Díez, M., Rosell, A. & Gil, D. (2015). Towards On-line Quantification of Tracheal Stenosis from Videobronchoscopy. International Journal of Computer Assisted Radiology and Surgery, 10(6), pp. 935-945. DOI: 10.1007/s11548-015-1196-z

[31] Krishnan, S. M., Yang, X., Chan, K. L., Kumar, S., & Goh, P. M. Y. (1998). Intestinal abnormality detection from endoscopic images. In Engineering in Medicine and Biology Society, 1998. Proceedings of the 20th Annual International Conference of the IEEE (Vol. 2, pp. 895-898). IEEE. DOI:10.1109/IEMBS.1998.745583

[32] Zhu, H., Fan, Y., & Liang, Z. (2011). Improved curvature estimation for shape analysis in computer-aided detection of colonic polyps. In Virtual Colonoscopy and Ab-

dominal Imaging. Computational Challenges and Clinical Opportunities (pp. 9-14). Springer Berlin Heidelberg. DOI: 10.1007/978-3-642-25719-3_2

[33] Tajbakhsh, N., Gurudu, S. R., & Liang, J. (2014). Automatic Polyp Detection Using Global Geometric Constraints and Local Intensity Variation Patterns. In Medical Image Computing and Computer-Assisted Intervention–MICCAI 2014(pp. 179-187). Springer International Publishing. DOI: 10.1007/978-3-319-10470-6_23

[34] Kang, J., & Doraiswami, R. (2003, May). Real-time image processing system for endoscopic applications. In Electrical and Computer Engineering, 2003. IEEE CCECE 2003. Canadian Conference on (Vol. 3, pp. 1469-1472). IEEE. DOI:10.1109/CCECE. 2003.1226181

[35] Burrus, C. S., Gopinath, R. A., & Guo, H. (1998). Introduction to wavelets and wavelet transforms (Vol. 998). New Jersey: Prentice hall.

[36] Bernal, J., Sánchez, F. J., & Vilariño, F. (2010). Feature Detectors and Feature Descriptors: Where We Are Now. Technical Report. Computer Vision Center.

[37] Ameling, S., Wirth, S., Paulus, D., Lacey, G., & Vilariño, F. (2009). Texture-based polyp detection in colonoscopy. In Bildverarbeitung für die Medizin 2009(pp. 346-350). Springer Berlin Heidelberg. DOI: 10.1007/978-3-540-93860-6_70

[38] Coimbra, M. T., & Cunha, J. S. (2006). MPEG-7 visual descriptors—contributions for automated feature extraction in capsule endoscopy. Circuits and Systems for Video Technology, IEEE Transactions on, 16(5), 628-637. DOI:10.1109/TCSVT.2006.873158

[39] Park, S. Y., Sargent, D., Spofford, I., & Vosburgh, K. G. (2012). A colon video analysis framework for polyp detection. Biomedical Engineering, IEEE Transactions on, 59(5), pp. 1408-1418. DOI: 10.1109/TBME.2012.2188397

[40] Xu, Y. R., & Zhao, J. (2014). Segmentation of haustral folds and polyps on haustral folds in CT colonography using complementary geodesic distance transformation. Journal of Shanghai Jiaotong University (Science), 19, pp. 513-520. DOI: 10.1007/ s12204-014-1534-2

[41] Van Wijk, C., Van Ravesteijn, V. F., Vos, F. M., & Van Vliet, L. J. (2010). Detection and segmentation of colonic polyps on implicit isosurfaces by second principal curvature flow. Medical Imaging, IEEE Transactions on, 29(3), pp. 688-698. DOI: 10.1109/TMI. 2009.2031323

[42] Bernal, J., Núnez, J. M., Sánchez, F. J., & Vilariño, F. (2014). Polyp Segmentation Method in Colonoscopy Videos by Means of MSA-DOVA Energy Maps Calculation. In Clinical Image-Based Procedures. Translational Research in Medical Imaging (pp. 41-49). Springer International Publishing. DOI: 10.1007/978-3-319-13909-8_6

[43] Ganz, M., Yang, X., & Slabaugh, G. (2012). Automatic segmentation of polyps in colonoscopic narrow-band imaging data. Biomedical Engineering, IEEE Transactions on, 59(8), pp. 2144-2151. DOI: 10.1109/TBME.2012.2195314

[44] Bernal, J., Gil, D., Sánchez, C., & Sánchez, F. J. (2014). Discarding Non Informative Regions for Efficient Colonoscopy Image Analysis. In Computer-Assisted and Robotic Endoscopy (pp. 1-10). Springer International Publishing. DOI: 10.1007/978-3-319-13410-9_1

[45] Arnold, M. An Image Analysis and Machine Learning Approach to Measuring the Quality of Individual Colonoscopy Procedures, PhD Thesis, (2012).

[46] Tian, H., Srikanthan, T., & Asari, K. V. (2001). Automatic segmentation algorithm for the extraction of lumen region and boundary from endoscopic images. Medical and Biological Engineering and Computing, 39(1), pp. 8-14. DOI: 10.1007/BF02345260

[47] Lu, L., Zhang, D., Li, L., & Zhao, J. (2012). Fully automated colon segmentation for the computation of complete colon centerline in virtual colonoscopy. Biomedical Engineering, IEEE Transactions on, 59(4), pp. 996-1004. DOI:10.1109/TBME.2011.2182051

[48] Azzopardi, G., & Petkov, N. (2013). Automatic detection of vascular bifurcations in segmented retinal images using trainable COSFIRE filters. Pattern Recognition Letters, 34(8), pp. 922-933. DOI:10.1016/j.patrec.2012.11.002

[49] Pudzs, M., Fuksis, R., & Greitans, M. (2013, April). Palmprint image processing with non-halo complex matched filters for forensic data analysis. In Biometrics and Forensics (IWBF), 2013 International Workshop on (pp. 1-4). IEEE. DOI:10.1109/IWBF.2013.6547317

[50] Núñez, J. M., Bernal, J., Ferrer, M., & Vilariño, F. (2014). Impact of Keypoint Detection on Graph-Based Characterization of Blood Vessels in Colonoscopy Videos. In Computer-Assisted and Robotic Endoscopy (pp. 22-33). Springer International. DOI: 10.1007/978-3-319-13410-9_3

[51] Núñez, J. M., Bernal, J., Sánchez, F. J., & Vilariño, F. (2015). GRowing Algorithm for Intersection Detection (GRAID) in branching patterns. Machine Vision and Applications, 26(2-3), pp. 387-400. DOI: 10.1007/s00138-015-0663-4

[52] Julious, S. A. (2009). Sample sizes for clinical trials. CRC Press. DOI: 10.1201/9781584887409

[53] Abràmoff, M. D., Magalhães, P. J., & Ram, S. J. (2004). Image processing with ImageJ. Biophotonics international, 11(7), pp. 36-43.

[54] Chapelle, O., Haffner, P., & Vapnik, V. N. (1999). Support vector machines for histogram-based image classification. Neural Networks, IEEE Transactions on, 10(5), pp. 1055-1064. DOI:10.1109/72.788646